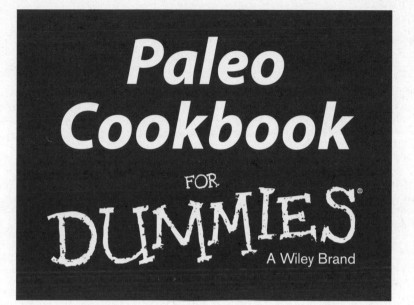

Paleo Cookbook

FOR DUMMIES®

A Wiley Brand

by Dr. Kellyann Petrucci

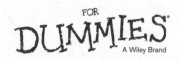

FOR DUMMIES®
A Wiley Brand

Paleo Cookbook For Dummies®

Published by: **John Wiley & Sons, Inc.,** 111 River Street, Hoboken, NJ 07030-5774, www.wiley.com

Copyright © 2013 by John Wiley & Sons, Inc., Hoboken, New Jersey

Media and software compilation copyright © 2013 by John Wiley & Sons, Inc. All rights reserved.

Published simultaneously in Canada

No part of this publication may be reproduced, stored in a retrieval system or transmitted in any form or by any means, electronic, mechanical, photocopying, recording, scanning or otherwise, except as permitted under Sections 107 or 108 of the 1976 United States Copyright Act, without the prior written permission of the Publisher. Requests to the Publisher for permission should be addressed to the Permissions Department, John Wiley & Sons, Inc., 111 River Street, Hoboken, NJ 07030, (201) 748-6011, fax (201) 748-6008, or online at http://www.wiley.com/go/permissions.

Trademarks: Wiley, For Dummies, the Dummies Man logo, Dummies.com, Making Everything Easier, and related trade dress are trademarks or registered trademarks of John Wiley & Sons, Inc., and may not be used without written permission. All other trademarks are the property of their respective owners. John Wiley & Sons, Inc., is not associated with any product or vendor mentioned in this book.

For general information on our other products and services, please contact our Customer Care Department within the U.S. at 877-762-2974, outside the U.S. at 317-572-3993, or fax 317-572-4002. For technical support, please visit www.wiley.com/techsupport.

Wiley publishes in a variety of print and electronic formats and by print-on-demand. Some material included with standard print versions of this book may not be included in e-books or in print-on-demand. If this book refers to media such as a CD or DVD that is not included in the version you purchased, you may download this material at http://booksupport.wiley.com. For more information about Wiley products, visit www.wiley.com.

Library of Congress Control Number: 2013938104

ISBN 978-1-118-61155-5 (pbk); ISBN 978-1-118-61138-8 (ebk); ISBN 978-1-118-61144-9 (ebk); ISBN 978-1-118-61156-2 (ebk)

Manufactured in the United States of America

10 9 8 7 6 5 4 3 2 1

Contents at a Glance

Recipes at a Glance

The following Paleo-approved recipes have been vetted by the team at Whole9 (http://whole9life.com) and are considered acceptable for a cleansing 30-day Paleo launch.

Table of Contents

Introduction

Any Paleo aficionado will agree that your Paleo journey starts with food. Discovering the yes and no Paleo foods, converting your kitchen into a primal one, and creating your own Paleo meals can help you lose weight, boost immunity, fight aging, heal conditions, and perform better.

Paleo recipes are a big hit for good reason. The food is amazing, and the recipes are easy to throw together. They work. Simple as that. Paleo recipes are all based on clean, ultra-healthy foods that are anything but boring. You don't feel like you're sacrificing; more importantly, you actually feel alive, vibrant, and nourished after you eat, not exhausted, bloated, and uncomfortable.

When I wrote this book, my vision was to give you something different. *Paleo Cookbook For Dummies* is unlike any other Paleo cookbook you've ever read. It's a collection of 136 recipes from the best of the best Paleo chefs out there. Each chef has his or her own creative flair, which adds a lot of variety to your recipe choices. These brilliantly created recipes will shock your friends and family when they find out that the food they're eating is actually super healthy!

I wrote this book to make your life simple. I have a busy life, and I'm sure you do too. I hope this easy-to-read, comprehensive book on Paleo foods and recipes makes your life easier. This book is also a great way for you to share your Paleo passion. In fact, next time you have a potluck, ask everyone to bring a recipe from this book, and prepare to be amazed!

About This Book

Getting back into the kitchen and adopting the Paleo diet may seem overwhelming at first, so *Paleo Cookbook For Dummies* is organized in a way that makes the benefits of eating Paleo easy to understand. Use this book as both a reference and a cookbook; if you need to check on whether a food is a Paleo yes or no, you can find that information easily. If you're creating a menu for a dinner party and want to go all Paleo, you can pick your recipes and get to work. Or if Paleo is new to you, you can start with the foundational information and get to know Paleo superfoods, how Paleo eating can improve how you feel, and how you can get started with a cleansing 30-Day Reset. And know that you can skip over the shaded sidebars and anything marked with a Technical Stuff icon if you're under a time crunch; these bits are interesting, but you won't miss out on any vital information if you pass them over.

The recipes in this book will keep you well fed from breakfast through dinner, with healthy snacks in between. Here are some specific recipe-related conventions that apply throughout the book:

- ♨ Vegetarian recipes are marked with a tomato in the Recipes in This Chapter list.

- ✔ Temperatures are all given in degrees Fahrenheit. (If you prefer working in the metric system, turn to the appendix for help converting temperatures to Celsius and other measurements to metric units.)

- ✔ All eggs are large unless noted otherwise.

- ✔ All water is filtered so all the toxic elements are removed.

- ✔ All bacon is free of nitrates, casein, gluten, and antibiotics.

- ✔ All pepper is freshly ground black pepper unless otherwise noted.

- ✔ All butter is grass-fed and organic. (If you can't find grass-fed butter, though, you can substitute conventional organic butter.) You may also replace any butter with *ghee* (clarified butter).

- ✔ All salt is unprocessed. Good sources for unprocessed salt include Selina Naturally brand Celtic sea salt (www.celticseasalt.com) and Real Salt brand sea salt (http://realsalt.com).

At the end of many recipes, you'll see a note indicating that the recipe has been vetted by the team at Whole9 (http://whole9life.com) and is considered acceptable for a cleansing 30-day Paleo launch, which I refer to in this book as the 30-Day Reset Paleo cleanse. These recipes don't include any added sugars (real or artificial), grains, legumes, or dairy. They replace butter with clarified butter (ghee). If a recipe includes a processed food (such as chicken broth, bacon, or tomato paste), you should choose brands that don't contain off-limits ingredients such as sugar, soy, additives, or preservatives.

To make this book practical as possible (because that's what it's really about, right?), I include web addresses for sources of products and other information. Some web addresses may break across two lines of text. If you're reading this book in print and want to visit one of these web pages, simply key in the address exactly as it's noted in the text, pretending as though the line break doesn't exist. If you're reading this text as an e-book, you've got it easy — just click the web address to be taken directly to the web page.

Foolish Assumptions

As I wrote this book, I made the following assumptions about you:

- ✔ You want to change your diet, lose weight, improve your fitness, or manage some type of medical condition and have heard about the Paleo diet.

- ✔ You want to stop eating processed and unhealthy foods to feel younger, healthier, happier, and more vibrant.

- ✔ You're open to the idea of making lifestyle changes — avoiding certain foods, making sleep a priority, reducing stress — to enhance your quality of life.

- ✔ You want to encourage yourself to continue the Paleo lifestyle by finding great-tasting recipes that are easy to make.

- ✔ You're adopting a level of commitment to Paleo that has you craving an all-around useful guidebook that has everything you could possibly need to jump back into your kitchen — and into your life.

- ✔ You have control over your food choices and those of your family, and you want to help your loved ones enjoy a healthy, Paleo lifestyle, too.

Icons Used in This Book

To make this book easier to navigate, I include the following icons to help you find key information about the Paleo lifestyle and Paleo cooking.

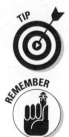

This icon indicates practical information that can help you in your quest for improving health, adopting a Paleo diet, or making one of the recipes.

When you see this icon, you know that the information that follows is important enough to read twice!

This icon highlights information that may be detrimental to your success if you ignore it.

This icon gives you a heads-up that what you're reading is more in-depth or technical than what you need to get a basic grasp on the main topic at hand.

Beyond the Book

In addition to all the material and recipes you can find in the book you're reading right now, this product also comes with some access-anywhere goodies on the web. Check out the eCheat Sheet at www.dummies.com/cheat sheet/paleocookbook for helpful insights and pointers on food principles you should and shouldn't follow for Paleo success, tips on using fats and spices, and some advice on food quality and snacking. You can also discover the ten biggest Paleo myths and how to bust them at www.dummies.com/extras/paleocookbook.

This book is packed with Paleo recipes — 136 of them, to be exact. But I couldn't stop there, so I include nine more tasty Paleo recipes online at www.dummies.com/extras/paleocookbook.

Where to Go from Here

This book is organized so you can read it in the way that makes the most sense to you; feel free to jump around to the information that's most relevant to you right now. You can use the table of contents to find the broad categories of subjects or use the index to look up specific information.

Do you want to know more about the Paleo superfoods so you can get started on the Paleo path? Start with Chapter 3. Ready to clean out your kitchen? Turn to Chapter 5. Feeling hungry and want to get started on the recipes? Feel free to jump right into the recipes in Parts II through IV.

If you're ready to detox your body with the Paleo lifestyle, you may want to jump right into the 30-Day Reset by reading Chapter 4. Chapter 6 provides an in depth look at where you can find Paleo foods.

And if you're not sure where to begin, read Part I. It gives you the basic information you need to understand why and how eating and living Paleo can help you improve your health and quality of life.

Part I
Exploring the Paleo Lifestyle

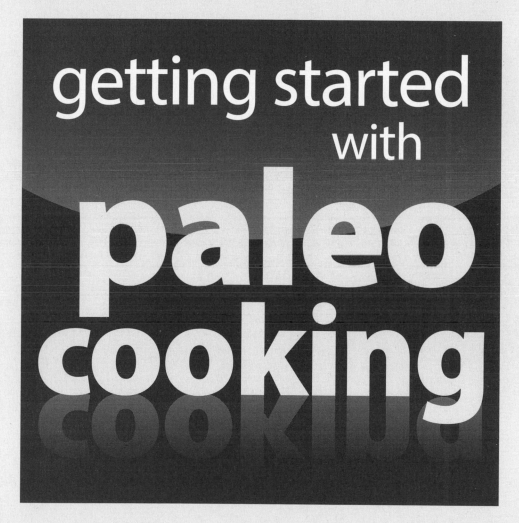

getting started
with
paleo
cooking

Visit www.dummies.com for free access to great Dummies content online.

In this part . . .

- Understand what makes Paleo a lifestyle (not just a diet) and how what happens outside the kitchen is as important as what happens inside.

- Load up on Paleo superfoods that give you the most bang for your buck to get you well and keep you well.

- Discover the power of detoxifying Paleo fruits and vegetables.

- Launch your Paleo lifestyle with a cleansing 30-Day Reset, which primes your body to achieve all the positive results of eating Paleo.

- Get advice on how to clean out and restock your kitchen with Paleo-approved foods.

Chapter 1

Becoming Paleo Smart

When I discovered the power of Paleo, my life changed, and I'm certainly not alone; Paleo has changed the lives of countless others as well. So much buzz surrounds Paleo because of its success in helping people lose weight, boost immunity, fight aging, heal conditions, and perform better. And who doesn't want to look and feel their best?

I wrote this book to help you discover the Paleo principles, getting you the best nutrition possible and showing you all the ins and outs on everything from what foods to buy (and what to toss) to where to get your food to how to cook the tastiest meals. The recipes you find in this book are from the absolute best Paleo culinary experts out there. All have different flairs and special touches to match your personal style. These recipes will entice you with their flavors and simplicity while providing you the best nutrition on the planet.

Paleo Cookbook For Dummies is your road map to the world of cooking and eating Paleo.

Surveying the Paleo Blueprint

The Paleo foods are your foundational foods — the foods your body is designed to have. The key concept behind Paleo is that nature determined what the human body needs before agriculture or modern food processing. In fact, DNA evidence shows that our genes have changed less than 0.02 percent in 40,000 years. Many of the foods that seem like common, everyday foods, such as grains, starchy carbohydrates, and drinks with sugar added, are really quite new compared to what was available when those genes were hard-wired.

My Paleo success story

I first became aware of the affects that food has on the body when I decided to do a fitness/bodybuilding contest in my 20s. In order to be contest-ready, I had to work with trainers on both my workouts and my nutrition.

The first tweak my trainer made to my diet was pulling out wheat/gluten. This approach wasn't at all a mainstream concept at that time like it is now. I and everyone around me were shocked at what happened to my body: I lost body fat, gained energy, and — what really surprised me — saw certain health conditions completely vanish.

Needless to say, I never went back to eating gluten again. I began eating what I thought was "clean" from then on, meaning I shopped only at natural health food stores and made sure everything I ate was organic and gluten-free. I continued to train regularly and followed my diet of "health foods."

This way of eating worked, until it didn't. As the years went on, I no longer got results. This shift was incredibly disheartening because I spent my life helping others with nutrition and made eating well an important part of my life. But I was at a crossroads. I could keep doing what I was doing and keep getting what I was getting, or I could find solutions. This desire led me on a path to find answers.

The solution I found seemed like an oversimplification. It wasn't a complicated program or a bunch of rules to follow short term. It was simply to *put real foods first*. To eat the foods with the highest *nutritional density* (high nutritional content relative to the calories it contains). Simple, back-to-nature foods that I was actually designed to have. When I did so, the magic happened. My body started de-aging and became fueled with energy; my eyes sparkled, and my skin glowed. It was as if my body was screaming out "I'm healthy!" I had no aches, pains, or conditions that were holding me back. As a clinician, I knew immediately that whatever was happening to me was happening on a deep, cellular level and that I needed to share this message of living Paleo with as many people as I could.

The foods on the Paleo plan are those that work best with your body. By really tuning into your body and your feelings about food, you start to instinctively become aware of which foods make you feel good and which don't.

Perusing Paleo foods in a nutshell

The Paleo diet is based on simple, easy-to-understand nutritional principles. What I love the most about eating Paleo is that it eliminates food confusion; it's simply about eating the foods that work best with your body.

Paleo-approved foods are whole, unprocessed foods: Meat, eggs, and seafood; non-starchy vegetables and Paleo-approved starchy vegetables; healthy fats; and some (but not a lot of) fruit, nuts, and seeds (see Figure 1-1).

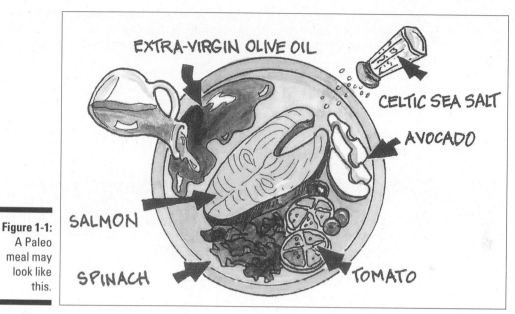

EXTRA-VIRGIN OLIVE OIL

CELTIC SEA SALT

AVOCADO

SALMON

SPINACH

TOMATO

Figure 1-1:
A Paleo
meal may
look like
this.

Illustration by Elizabeth Kurtzman

Paleo principles support avoiding foods with sugar, grains (even whole grains), legumes, and any processed, unhealthy oils. If you're going to be a straight-laced Paleo convert, then dairy's out because it can cause a host of problems for many people. However, some folks can enjoy some full-fat, organic, antibiotic-free dairy options (which seem to present less of a problem because of their source) like yogurt, *kefir* (a fermented dairy product), and *ghee* (clarified butter).

Think of it this way: If the food can be hunted or gathered, it's probably a safe bet. If the food has been processed or is presented to you in colorful, crinkly plastic packaging, it's probably a Paleo no-go.

Stick to the food choices that lead to optimal health in a modern world. You have to keep individual variation in mind. Some people may do okay on dairy; most others (about 80 percent) don't. Some can thrive on fewer carbohydrates; others need more. That's why eating a basic Paleo diet is the foundation; you adjust the basics in a way that works for your life.

Getting quick results by eating Paleo

I always say that if I had a football field full of patients and they told me what ailed them, the root of their problems would boil down to one of three sources: blood sugar problems, chronic inflammation, and gut disturbances. That's why so many health practitioners love Paleo: It provides the solution to these problems.

If you've been eating a lot of foods such as grains, processed foods, and sugars that have been causing inflammation, blood sugar problems, and gut irritation, you may just perk up in a flash. For some, that bloated feeling goes away after the first few meals.

Even if you don't currently have one of these ailments, know that all the nutrients in the Paleo-approved foods can really make you come alive, especially if you're coming from a place of nutrient deficiency. When you go from a state of deficiency to one of sufficiency, results can come pretty immediately.

Making Paleo work in your busy life

In modern-day life, speed seems to be the goal: How much can you get done in the shortest amount of time while trying to balance family and career? So the question becomes, how do you add one more layer — finding time to eat well and prepare meals — to this intensity?

In one way, you save time almost immediately because you're no longer aimless about what and where to eat. This sense of direction is pretty liberating. Shopping even becomes easy because you quickly learn exactly how to hunt and gather for Paleo foods (see Chapter 6 for more information on shopping).

You start developing food values; as a result, you become very clear on what you will and won't eat. Just like you go back to your moral values whenever you make a decision on anything —even if you aren't aware of it — you refer to your food values when making eating decisions. When you get into eating Paleo, you get a solid understanding of what works for you and what doesn't.

You can find other tips throughout this book on becoming organized and reallocating some of your time to help Paleo fit into your world. For example, *batch cooking* (preparing several days' worth of staple or convenience foods at once, such as hard-boiling eggs, precooking meats, and cutting and chopping veggies) saves a tremendous amount of time. After you get the hang of batch cooking, you get really fast and it becomes no big deal.

You can make eating Paleo practical in the modern world; in time, this lifestyle will become second nature to you.

I started a Paleo meal delivery service for folks who need just a little extra help having Paleo meals at the ready. Go to www.livingpaleofoods.com for more info on how you can get grass-fed, wild, organic prepared Paleo foods delivered right to your door! All meals are made with the highest food quality and cooked in the healthiest way. You just heat and eat.

Paleo success story: Krystle

I initially started living Paleo to help get rid of the last five to ten pounds that I had left to lose from being pregnant and nursing my daughter, who is now a year old. As I was starting to eat real foods, we found out that I was pregnant again with our second baby! I'm a pregnant, working mom and wife, and I find it important to have dinner ready when my family gets home so we can spend quality time together. Cooking a 20-to-30-minute meal is so easy by quickly steaming vegetables and preparing a salad while baking fish or chicken in the oven. Even a simple stir fry is so quick and delicious. I actually find cooking Paleo meals to be easier than any other kinds of foods.

I've cut my grocery shopping and cooking time by planning out my family's meals and snacks and being sure to only shop for the foods that are on that list. Knowing what the Paleo foods are makes shopping so easy because I'm not floundering around in the grocery store wondering what I should buy. If you're hesitant to try Paleo because you fear you don't have time, don't worry! Cooking Paleo will take you no more time (even less) than preparing traditional meals, and you'll look and feel so much better! I know I'm being a good role model for my family and helping them all to be healthy as possible. It feels good to be Paleo!

Reaping the Rewards of a Paleo Diet

Paleo often has a reputation for having magic effects because its benefits are so powerful for so many. The backbone of Paleo is really about getting you healthy. Everything in life rises and falls on your health, so when you get healthy, everything else falls into place.

Being healthy means giving your body the right raw materials so they can flourish. This raw material goes beyond eating certain foods to truly embracing a lifestyle — paying attention to why and how you eat and to other factors such as the amount and quality of your sleep, your stress levels, your sunlight intake, your movement level, and your thoughts. When you really go Paleo, you get lasting positive consequences, and the magic unfolds.

How long feeling this switch go on takes is different for everyone. For some, it's immediate; for others, it's a few days or maybe a few weeks. But if you stick to Paleo, it will go on for you, so hang tight!

Most people get started on Paleo to lose weight, but they end up getting more in return: reduced inflammation, lower blood sugar, better sleep, and cleared-up skin and gut issues, all of which I cover in the following sections.

Losing weight and looking younger

Losing weight happens because your body recalibrates or resets to a healthy weight. You lose stored fat because you actually use that stored fat for energy, making you lean and strong.

Here are five reasons you lose weight with Paleo foods:

✔ Where there is waste, there is weight. When your body has a lot of toxins, it naturally harbors more fat as a protective mechanism to store the toxins and protect your organs from them. When you're toxic, you're tired, sluggish, and much less active than you'd normally be. Therefore, the fewer toxins you have in your body, the healthier you are, and a healthy body stands the best chance of losing weight and burning fat. Paleo foods aren't refined and processed; therefore, they're very low in toxins. You're eating *nutrient dense* foods, which are filled with nutrition without all the toxic calories and additives

✔ Inflammation leaves the body, so that bloated, puffy look disappears. When this puffiness disappears, your intracellular and extracellular water balances in your system; you lose that extra water weight and begin to get a lean, healthy look.

✔ Many suffer from weight loss resistance because of food sensitivities. The Paleo foods are low-allergen foods, so they cause fewer sensitivities and associated weight issues.

✔ Paleo foods help you maintain a healthy blood sugar, so you're less likely to get that so-called muffin top around your waist.

✔ You achieve your body's *set point* (the weight set by your genetics at which your body naturally tries to settle) by eating foods that regulate your hormones along with the signals associated with hormones.

Paleo success story: Noel

Noel started eating Paleo for one reason: She wanted to lose that "freshman 15." She lost the 15 pounds with ease and was surprised at all the other benefits that came with eating Paleo. Noel says, "I focus better than ever, so I know it has made me a better student. I also didn't realize that the refined carbs and dairy were making me feel so bloated and heavy and were the cause of all my stomach problems. I have lots of energy to work out now, whereas before I was too run-down — and my skin looks so much better. I'm so thankful for discovering *Living Paleo For Dummies* (Wiley) and am thrilled to hear about the accompanying cookbook! I love the Paleo lifestyle, and my sister and I are having a ball making Paleo recipes. This college girl is definitely Paleo for life!"

Clearing up gut and skin issues

Beauty really is an inside job. What you see on your face is a mirror image of what's happening on the inside, and when your intestines are damaged, it shows.

What causes this damage is typical modern-day lifestyle patterns. Many modern foods lack nutrients and fiber, are filled with toxins, and don't have the healthy bacteria you need to create healthy intestinal cells. If you have acne, rashes, eczema, psoriasis, poor skin tone, and so on, *leaky gut* (where the cells of your small intestine lose their integrity and become porous, creating inflammation and havoc in your body) may be the problem.

Here are some of the offenders in this typical scenario of leaky gut:

- ✔ Grains, including whole grains and grain-like seeds such as wheat, barley, oats, spelt, brown rice, quinoa, and corn
- ✔ Beans and legumes
- ✔ Anti-inflammatory medications (NSAIDS)
- ✔ Refined foods
- ✔ Alcohol
- ✔ Sugar
- ✔ Dairy
- ✔ Poor-quality fats and oils

If you've consumed any of these items over the years, you may be facing a problem of leaky gut.

The good news is that this condition can be reversed fairly easily. Paleo creates healthier intestinal cells. Eating the nutrient-rich Paleo foods helps heal your intestinal lining, which makes your skin look beautiful and keeps you well. Avoiding the offenders and sticking to Paleo foods infuses your body with good nutrients and bacteria to heal your gut. (Flip to Chapter 3 for information on choosing Paleo foods.)

For additional healing nutrients for your gut, make sure you eat foods such as raw sauerkraut and kimchi, which provide good bacteria, and foods such as sweet potatoes and butternut squash, which contain good soluble fiber. If you have an illness you're trying to reverse or a stubborn skin condition that you suspect stems from leaky gut, you may want to remove eggs, coffee, nuts, and seeds as well until your gut has time to heal. You may even want to consider supplementing with a probiotic in a pill or powder form.

Paleo success story: Julie

Living Paleo and loving it! I decided to go Paleo and take the family with me. I gave them no choice after hearing Dr. Kellyann speak — and they're thanking me now.

What convinced me I really needed to take the plunge was my psoriasis. What I didn't expect was that after the first week, my entire family felt better, and we couldn't believe the food we ate had such an impact. Best of all, no one was hungry. My husband and I both lost at least five pounds immediately, and that was a welcome bonus. We made our weekly menu like we always did with a few adjustments. I have to admit the Paleo recipes were a needed change. I quickly learned what meals were good for weeknights and what needed to be made on the weekend. My psoriasis is now markedly improved in only eight short weeks, and I can't tell you how exciting it is to see those changes in my body! I've suffered with this condition for so long. I loved the weight loss, the clear skin, and most of all the energy I have. My family didn't miss a beat, and we are all better for it! Eight weeks now, and well on our way to what I call the Paleo lifestyle!

Sleeping better

Better sleep is my motivation behind sticking as closely as I can to the Paleo foods. All Paleo followers have a personal Paleo barometer that tells them when they've gotten too far off track and need to pull back and reset their bodies with strictly Paleo foods. For some, it's pains or weight gain, but for me, it's sleep. If I go off the rails too much, my sleep suffers, and I know that it's time to pull back. I actually know many folks who fell in love with Paleo when they discovered it would make them sleep better.

Here are some reasons Paleo helps you sleep like a baby:

- Paleo foods are packed with minerals, a great natural sleep aid.
- Balanced blood sugar causes fewer sleep disturbances.
- Eating Paleo helps balance your hormones and signals associated with hormones to provide a feeling of stability and calm, which helps you feel better and thus sleep better.

Some additional tips to get better sleep include making sure you avoid all sweeteners (including artificial and Paleo-approved natural sweeteners) as well as caffeine because they can really cause blood sugar disturbances, which in turn affect sleep. After you have avoided sweeteners long enough to reset your body and are able to sleep naturally, you can add some Paleo-approved sweeteners such as honey back into your diet. Keep in mind that alcohol, stress, and chronic exercise (overtraining) all can negatively impact sleep, too.

Balancing your blood sugar

If you have problems maintaining your blood sugar, eating Paleo foods (and the recipes in this book) is a great place for you to get the help you need to move toward health. Yes, Paleo can even improve/heal blood sugar problems.

When you eat a well-balanced Paleo meal of lean meats, Paleo-approved carbohydrates, and healthy fats, you don't have all those blood sugar swings that you once had. Your body is no longer forced to constantly release insulin, and your blood sugar stabilizes.

Consider Drew, a 56-year-old horticulturist whose blood sugar went from 358 down to the 90–100 range in just four months of strict Paleo (see Figure 1-2). His story has inspired many to give Paleo a shot.

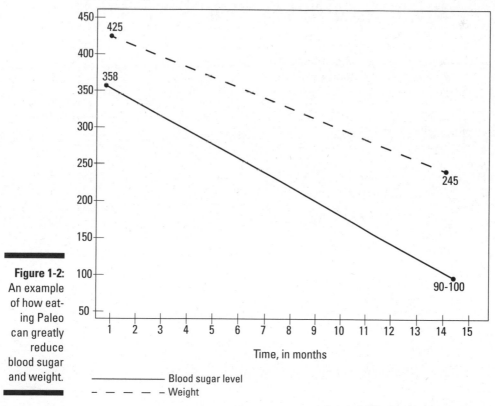

Figure 1-2: An example of how eating Paleo can greatly reduce blood sugar and weight.

Illustration by Wiley, Composition Services Graphics

Paleo success story: John

John noticed that his vision began to get a bit blurry and he couldn't see as well as he had. This change prompted a checkup that revealed he had a blood sugar of 220, much higher than the normal range of about 90 to 120. He began eating Paleo foods, and his blood sugars plummeted to approximately 115! His vision sharpened, and he could see clearly once again. He was surprised to find himself feeling more energized (he said he was always lethargic before); he felt stronger — as if his muscle mass was improving. He also found himself healing much more quickly.

John's story is a perfect example of the healing effects of Paleo. When you allow your body to get truly healthy, it has a domino effect on all of the structures and functions of the body!

Reducing inflammation

A lot of the problems people have today are caused by inflammation in the body. Short-term inflammation is actually a part of a normal healing process. When your immune system overreacts and shifts into high gear, that's when you have a problem known as *chronic inflammation*.

Here are some of the conditions associated with chronic inflammation:

- ✔ Acne
- ✔ Arthritis
- ✔ Asthma and allergies
- ✔ Celiac disease
- ✔ Colitis
- ✔ Crohn's disease
- ✔ Eczema
- ✔ Inflammatory bowel disease (IBD)
- ✔ Leaky gut
- ✔ Migraines
- ✔ Multiple sclerosis (MS)
- ✔ PCOS
- ✔ Thyroid disorders
- ✔ Ulcerative colitis

When you begin eating Paleo foods, you kick to the curb a lot of the processed foods and grains that cause this inflammation. Paleo foods are by nature anti-inflammatory and keep your immune system strong, so you effectively prevent and heal inflammatory conditions.

 Make sure you're not just eating Paleo but also living Paleo. Exposure to toxins, stress, medications, overtraining, and sleep deprivation can all affect inflammation.

Undergoing the Paleo Transformation

You live longer, stronger, and more healthfully when you start eating and living Paleo because you move toward health. When you're truly healthy, your immune system is solid, protective, and strong. Your body works for you, not against you, and transformation happens.

I love to see what I call *the Paleo transformation*. People usually start Paleo to lose weight. Then layers and layers begin to peel back. Their waists get smaller, their skin and eyes glisten, and their hair may get shinier. They notice conditions healing, and before long, they get the most amazing part of the transformation — a mental, spiritual kind of change. They start thinking more clearly and enjoying a more positive outlook. When I see this start to unfold in the Paleo progression, I know healing is happening on the deepest level. I always call it "watching the de-aging process" because eating Paleo reboots the body by flooding it with vitamins and minerals. This healing is possible for anyone who decides to commit to living Paleo!

Choosing health with the Paleo Manifesto

To really look and feel your best for life, the Paleo principles are a template that works. Keep in mind the following tenets, which are woven throughout living Paleo:

Our bodies are really an energy matrix, and we should think of ourselves as electrical beings, not just structural ones. We are atoms and molecules, not just skin and bones.

Your genes express themselves according to your lifestyle. The way you eat, move, and live has everything to do with the outcome of your health. Living in a way that most closely matches your blueprint is most congruent with health and happiness. Finding time to play, get sunshine, exercise, connect with others, disconnect from electronics, and manage your stress all matter.

Most importantly, health is a byproduct of your choices. Living and eating Paleo is the healthiest template I have seen in all of my years of practice and helping people and other doctors find solutions. Results are typical with living Paleo.

Identifying why Paleo works better than other approaches

Paleo is more effective than other approaches because it centers on the food that works best with your body. Most importantly, Paleo foods have one purpose, which is what truly defines Paleo: to nourish the body and get you healthy.

That's right, the objective behind eating Paleo is to get you healthy. Period. Everything else that comes along the way just follows the natural progression. It's against natural law not to lose weight, boost immunity, fight aging, heal conditions, and perform better when you're healthy.

Switching on your healthy genes with Paleo

You're in the driver's seat of your health. Your lifestyle choices and the environment in which you choose to live have the biggest impact on the quality of your life. This science is called *epigenetics*. If you feel as though you can't lose weight or get well, no matter how much Paleo food you eat, because of your genes, you can erase all that thinking. Epigenetics is proof that how we look and feel is the result of our choices. Think of epigenetics as your ambassador of health. Epigenetics sends messages to your genome (genes) telling it to flick on the switch of health — or not — depending on your lifestyle choices.

If you're living Paleo, your body will flip the switch to health, and your genes will express this choice. You'll be healthy, lean, strong, and energetic. If you aren't making healthy choices, your genes will express sickness, fatigue, or obesity.

A Paleo diet and lifestyle create the raw material your genes need to flip the switch to health. You find that you look and feel your best — naturally.

Have a Paleo party

If you want to enroll others in living Paleo, start by having a Paleo party! Ask everyone to bring a recipe from this book. Discussing what's in some of the dishes is fun, and when your guests taste Paleo food for themselves, they're intrigued by how good it is with healthy Paleo ingredients. It's a fun and enlightening way to get people loving Paleo. My sister and I did this kind of event one New Year's Eve to celebrate the launch of *Living Paleo For Dummies* (Wiley), and it was an absolute blast.

Chapter 2

Creating a Paleo Lifestyle

*E*ating Paleo foods is exciting. It's a simple approach to eating that has gained so much traction in mainstream media because of its landmark success in helping people lose weight and get healthy. But that's just the beginning of the story.

Paleo is a lifestyle, not a flash-in-the-pan, red-carpet diet with the entire focus on just getting the weight off. That's the magic of Paleo: It does get the weight off, but it does so by creating healthier cells. When you create healthier cells, you naturally lose weight, boost your immunity, heal your body, and fight aging. You literally get healthier from the inside out when you live a Paleo lifestyle. It's against natural law not to.

Putting real food first is the foundation. However, Paleo considers all influences on your body, even those that happen outside the kitchen. Your relationship with food and how your food makes you feel, how much you eat, your movement, your exposure to sunlight, supplementation, your stress levels, and your thoughts all matter. Each of these variables creates the building blocks for the positive, long-lasting effects of living Paleo.

Ultimately, your habits and patterns are the defining factor of your success in losing weight, healing your body, boosting your immunity, and aging gracefully. This chapter gives you the lifestyle strategies that have positive lasting effects, allowing you to live your life by the optimal design shaped and molded by nature.

Getting an Overview of Living Paleo

One of the major beliefs in today's society is that the best way to lose weight and feel better is through whatever diet sheds the fat the fastest and whatever pill takes your symptoms away the quickest. Stop for a minute and ask yourself, "How's this working out?"

People are fatter and sicker than ever. Chronic diseases such as heart disease, diabetes, and cancer are affecting more people than ever. If modern-day living was evaluated like most businesses are, it would be considered a business model that needs improving, if not complete restructuring.

Here's the good news. You have a blueprint that works right at your fingertips. It's called *living Paleo*. When you discover the strategies for living how you were designed to eat, move, think, and live, a better life unfolds. Your life takes on a healthier, happier rhythm, and you flourish in every way. The best part is that it all happens naturally, as if your body was made for this lifestyle all along!

Seeing Paleo as more than a diet

Most people start eating Paleo because they know someone (or someone who knows someone) who is getting awesome results — they're losing weight, feeling great, and looking healthier and better than ever. Getting a killer body is pretty great incentive, no doubt. But these effects are just the tip of the iceberg.

The Paleo lifestyle isn't just a diet; it's a life-improvement framework that gets results. You can set your watch to it. After you start putting real foods such as healthy proteins, fats, and carbohydrates into your body, you flourish in every way, not just on the scale. You have the energy to look for ways to heal on a deeper level. You move more, sleep better, spend more time outdoors, are more social, and even feel more optimistic. (I discuss several of these aspects of the lifestyle throughout this chapter.)

When you adopt the Paleo lifestyle patterns, you say goodbye to illness, aches, pains, and fatigue. You lose excess weight, and inflammation and bloating disappear. You start to look and feel younger. You're bursting with energy, and enthusiasm floods back into your life.

Shifting your belief system

Wrapping your head around Paleo living means changing your belief system, or *paradigm*. You may be used to some of the following beliefs about eating, which Paleo debunks:

- ✔ Cow's milk is the best way to get your calcium.
- ✔ Beans offer the benefits of superimmunity and fiber.
- ✔ Grains and whole grains are an essential part of a healthy diet.
- ✔ Soy is a superfood.
- ✔ A slab of meat and a baked potato make up the perfect meal.
- ✔ If you want to balance your blood sugar, grab a cheese stick.
- ✔ Fruit is healthy, so eat as much as you want.
- ✔ Red meat is really bad for you and will make your heart explode.
- ✔ Fat is evil.
- ✔ You should eat eggs in strict moderation because they raise your cholesterol.
- ✔ Vegetarian-based diets are the healthiest.

These statements may have been a big part of your life, so the Paleo principles may take you by surprise. Until of course, you see the cold hard truth: the undisputable results.

The question becomes will you make the paradigm changes necessary to live your healthiest life? Some people may need to make only small changes, but others may need to make bigger changes. Shifting your belief system requires a conscious choice to embrace health. Your choices determine your health, not bad genes or bad luck.

Adjusting your belief system so that you constantly work toward choosing health may be one of the best gifts you can give yourself. When your body gets the raw material it requires to function at its best, the magic starts to happen.

Considering the living Paleo solution versus modern medicine

In 2004, Former Surgeon General of the United States Dr. Richard Carmona stated, "Because of the increasing rates of obesity, unhealthy eating habits, and physical inactivity, we may see the first generation that will be less healthy and have a shorter life expectancy than their parents." That's an unbelievable statement: that U.S. children today will be the first generation to not outlive their parents simply because of lifestyle choices!

Modern medicine isn't the answer. All the modern drugs and surgeries clearly aren't making the population well or improving lives. The United States spends about $1.4 trillion annually on the supposed health care system, but studies show about one-third of medical spending is now devoted to services that don't improve the quality of care. In fact, in some cases treatment may even make your overall condition worse.

A lot of what falls under the heading of health care is really more like sickness care. Drugs were never designed to get patients healthier. They were designed to get them out of crisis mode, not to move them toward health. And taking medications does nothing to change behavior. If you want health, that job is up to you. No shortcut or magic pill can do it for you. Only the lifestyle you choose to live can. Don't let modern medicine give you permission to lead a life that doesn't serve you.

You have to be a participant in your healing to get results. Discovering the right paradigm and making smart choices go a long way in helping you lose weight, heal your body, boost immunity, and fight aging.

Following Basic Rules for the Paleo Lifestyle

When patients come to me for nutritional consultation — whether they want to heal themselves of something or lose weight — I want to know about their lifestyle patterns right off the bat. That's the treasure map. When I learn how they eat, move, think, and live their daily lives, the pieces to the puzzle of why they don't look and feel as amazing as they should start falling into place.

Your habits create your destiny, and that plays out profoundly in your physiology. Like it or not, the human body is designed to live a certain way, and the more we stray from nature's blueprint, the more we suffer. The environment you choose to live in and stay in determines whether you create a healthy body or an unhealthy body, so choose an environment that lets your body function the way it was designed. The following sections point out a few major guidelines for creating a Paleo-conducive environment (don't worry; none of them involves moving to a cave).

Sticking to the 80-percent rule

To get long-lasting results, you can benefit from spending at least 30 days eating a strict Paleo diet (flip to Chapter 4 for details on this Paleo cleanse). After that, the 80-percent rule keeps you in check both physically and health-wise. The *80-percent rule* means that if you adhere to Paleo principles at least 80 percent of the time, you'll experience the benefits of Paleo. If you eat poorly, you'll feel bad. What you eat is like the foundation of a house, and you must build a healthy framework to build a solid house. That said, you do have a little life leeway; you can adjust the rule to fit your personal needs.

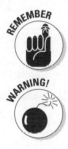

This 80-percent rule assumes that you're not trying to heal yourself of an illness or lose considerable weight. If you are, you may need to be 90 percent compliant or more for a while.

The 80-percent rule isn't a license to fill 20 percent of your diet with crummy processed foods or go to town on cookies, pancakes, bread, or muffins — even if they're Paleo! Sugar is still sugar, and too much of it is going to send you right back to needing a 30-day Paleo cleanse.

Some people choose to eat Paleo 90 or even 100 percent of the time, which is very powerful. Others feel that eating Paleo even 80 percent of the time causes constant cravings. It really comes down to food choices and what works best for you in your life.

Increasing the amount and quality of sleep you get

Quality sleep is what's essential for losing weight or being healthy. One of the most priceless factors when eating and living a healthy lifestyle is improvement to your sleep cycle. After your body adjusts to eating cleaner, more nutrient-dense foods, you find your sleep is deeper and more restful. One of my personal motivations for living Paleo is it helps me get restful sleep. It really does make a tremendous difference.

Think about living by your body's design. Your hunter-gatherer ancestors naturally dozed off when the fire went out at the end of an evening. They didn't have a light switch or pill to keep them up. They trudged along their day, and when their meal and socializing were over, the flames blew out and they naturally went to sleep.

Not getting quality sleep is one of the more common frustrations of patients. Maybe you have trouble falling asleep, or you wake in the middle of the night, unable to drift back to sleep. No matter what the scenario, eating Paleo foods completely changes the quality and duration of your sleep. Here are some of the reasons this shift happens:

- ✔ You're getting foods loaded with minerals, which is grounding and calming to your body.

- ✔ Your blood sugar is more balanced, so you don't get that blood sugar dip in the middle of the night that causes your body to release hormones and disturbs sleep.

- ✔ Healthy foods contain B vitamins, which are great for calming nerves and balancing the nervous system for restful sleep.

- ✔ Some of the Paleo foods like eggs, turkey, nuts, fish, and some fruits contain an essential amino acid called *tryptophan* that helps promote sleep.

- ✔ When eating foods with superior nutrition, your body naturally regulates hormones and signals associated with hormones that in turn help you sleep better.

If you feel you need a little help sleeping until all the structures and functions of your body regulate and heal, try Natural Calm (`http://naturalvitality.com/natural-calm`). It's a great natural magnesium supplement that may help you sleep a little better.

Becoming more social

Are you an introvert or an extrovert? The real definition of these terms may be different than what you have in mind. An *introvert* is someone who gets fatigued when she's around people for an extended period and often needs time away to recharge. On the other hand, an *extrovert* finds being around people exhilarating, and that recharges her in and of itself. Extroverts feel no need to have some alone time.

Is sleep really overrated?

Why should you care so much about getting good sleep? Here are the top four motivators to convince you to turn off the TV or shut down the computer and get some shut-eye:

✔ **Cancer:** Not getting enough sleep doubles your risk of breast cancer.

✔ **Weight gain:** Sleep deprivation causes you to gain weight; proper sleep causes you to lose weight. You can lose 14.3 pounds a year by getting one more hour of sleep per night.

✔ **Earlier death:** In 2004, a study in the journal *Sleep* found that women who averaged less than five hours of sleep per night had a higher death rate than those who slept seven hours.

✔ **Insulin resistance and heart disease:** When you don't get enough sleep, hormones shift, causing your appetite to change. The sugars you crave shoot your insulin up and create blood sugar problems, which cause weight gain and health issues such as insulin resistance. *Insulin resistance* causes you to convert all your carbohydrates into bad cholesterol, which can cause heart related diseases as well.

No matter where you fall on the social spectrum, one thing is for certain: Your body is healthiest when you take some time out to be a part of a community or socialize. Humans aren't designed to be alone for an extended period. Your social blueprint is wired to spend time around others, enjoying yourself. Your hunter-gatherer ancestors travelled together in bands and socialized every night by the fire. They played, sang, danced, or just shared stories (maybe about the day's kill or the berries that were foraged).

Although some time alone is definitely beneficial, be sure to actively include social time as another path to wellness. Joining a community or group of people with like-minded interests can really make a difference in your life. I make it a point to be in programs or groups with people who are writers, health care providers, or entrepreneurs because I understand that deep down, doing so is as important to my health as anything else I do.

You make be thinking, "But I'm busy enough already!" I get it, believe me. Especially when you still have young children at home. Just remember that you're better at everything else you do when you satisfy your soul's innate desire for connection!

Finding ways to eat Paleo at dinner parties

Socializing is fun, and you need to socialize to be happy, so try to work with other people's lifestyles while holding firm on your own food values. If you have the ability to ask what will be served, that's great. But in most cases, you have to just deal. You can't make a fuss about it unless the host or hostess makes a point to ask ahead whether guests have any dietary concerns — which I'm finding happens more and more these days. If you *are* asked, you shouldn't launch into some kind of Paleo scroll, like "Well, please omit grains, dairy, legumes, and, oh, no soy please." You may be scratched off that dinner party list — permanently!

If you are asked for dietary requests, mention that baked or grilled protein with some vegetables would be really great, and that sauces can be problematic for you, so just some herbs and spices will do the trick perfectly.

What I've always done is bring my own Paleo dish to share. The host/hostess usually loves the idea of a backup dish, and the contribution opens the door to conversation about Paleo and maybe even some converts. "Paleo, what's that? Boy, this is delicious."

Spending time outdoors

One of the most important shifts in your health is to spend time outdoors so that you get sunshine. When sunlight hits the skin, a process begins that leads to the creation and activation of vitamin D. Your hunter-gather ancestors spent a lot of time outdoors. The sunlight provided them with health and vibrancy.

To make radical changes in your future health, be clear about this point: Sunlight is a nutrient. When your body creates vitamin D, your body fights colds and the flu better as well as osteoporosis, cancer, heart disease, depression, and a host of other conditions. When you're outdoors getting sun and vitamin D, your body also produces more of the feel-good hormone serotonin, which helps you relax.

Regular sun exposure is grossly understated as a vitally important barrier to disease. You may worry about sun-related skin damage and skin cancers, but intermittent exposure actually increases your odds because you have a great chance of burning, and burning is what cause your risk factors to go up. Regular exposure to the sun protects against skin cancers.

How much exposure you need to get your dose of vitamin D depends on how dark your skin is and environmental factors such as how close you live to the equator or what time of day you're in the sun. It's usually about 20 minutes daily of sunshine for the average person at peak times. The darker your skin, the more exposure you need.

Start practicing the *slow immersion* process without sunscreen so you can benefit from vitamin D. When you get frequent short periods of exposure, you build a protective layer. Build up your tolerance on a regular basis, gradually and early in the spring to prep your skin for the stronger summer sun. Try to get sun earlier in the morning where you have less chance of burning and overheating.

When you do need sunscreen, the Environmental Working Group's Skin Deep website (www.ewg.org/skindeep) can help you find the best natural, non-toxic sunscreen.

Spending more time outdoors has so many benefits. Chances are that if you're spending more time outdoors, you're moving your body more and spending less time in front of the television or computer. You may even be fitting in more time for play. These changes alone can improve your health.

Reprogramming your mindset

How you think (or as my dad would always say, "the six inches between your ears") is really what defines you. Understanding your mindset is essential if you want to embrace wellness.

Major influences in your life — whether they're your parents, teachers, preachers, or whatever — programmed your current belief systems, which in turn create your reality. In fact, most of your programming (your unconscious thought) is wired in your brain by the time you're 18. Here's where it gets really interesting: Your unconscious mind is responsible for about 95 percent of your thoughts during the course of a day. Therefore, the programming you received as a youngster is still guiding you through life today.

You may not have had any say in how you were programmed when you were younger, but you do now! You can reprogram your thoughts to be healthier and more positive. Having positive thoughts is an essential piece of living healthfully and aging well.

One the best ways to reprogram your mind is through using positive *affirmations* (statements of conviction) and journaling. You have to override all the negative affirmations that you replay in your mind by repeating your positive affirmations over and over. You begin to become aware that you really do create your reality. Start by journaling your affirmations in a notebook and saying them out loud in the morning (before your mind has time to fight back). Use the present tense as if your affirmations were already happening, such as "I AM lean, strong, and healthy, and every day I'm creating what I want." Say them with intention and with complete clarity — don't rush through them. Write and say your affirmations over and over until your physiology believes you. Soon your affirmations will become part of you!

Eating Paleo when eating out

Eating Paleo doesn't mean you have to be perfect. When you eat out, it's up to you how much leeway you give yourself. Some people may be very reactive to certain foods and have to be very careful, but maybe a little traditional salad dressing or some sushi with white rice works for you. The point is to always be aware of how certain foods make you feel. If you feel sick, tired, bloated, cranky, constipated, or otherwise upset digestively, that's your call to stay away.

To prepare for your dining experience,

- ✔ Always call ahead to ask questions or for special requests.

- ✔ Look for the menus online and plan ahead.

- ✔ Beware of the starters like the bread baskets and chips. They are usually filled with non-Paleo foods. If your dining companions don't mind, don't let the server even bring these freebies to the table, or have them remove the pre-set baskets.

When reviewing the menu, avoid foods that are described as "battered," "breaded," "coated," "crispy," "deep-fried," or "fritter." These designations usually mean unhealthy oils and cooking methods were used.

If your restaurant choice offers ethnic cuisine, here are some tips:

- ✔ **Mexican:** Stick to meat, salsa, and guacamole. If you like tacos or fajitas, eat just the filling and skip the shells.

- ✔ **Italian:** Choose chicken, beef, and fish dishes. Look for sautéed or grilled vegetables that you can order with garlic and olive oil or red sauce. I always opt for the antipasto platter dressed in olive oil.

- ✔ **Thai:** Curry dishes are typically loaded with protein, coconut milk, and vegetables, which are all good.

- ✔ **Indian:** I always go for the tandoori dishes, which are cooked in the tandoori oven. Ask whether other dishes are cooked with flour or yogurt, and if so, avoid them.

- ✔ **Japanese:** Order maki or hand rolls and ask that they be made without rice. Sashimi is another excellent option, and you can round off your meal with a seaweed salad. If you like to use soy sauce, bring your own bottle of coconut aminos to substitute.

- ✔ **Greek:** Roasted chicken, kebabs, grilled fish, and Greek salad without the feta cheese all work nicely. The olives are fantastic too.

- ✔ **Middle Eastern:** Stick to lamb, beef, pork, vegetables, and chicken shawarma. The *baba gannoujh* (pureed eggplant) or tahini (sesame seed paste) are Middle Eastern favorites and Paleo all the way.

Taking a technology timeout

Computers, smartphones, and other handheld devices are super convenient (I for one love my computer and cellphone), but shutting down once in a while is important — your cells benefit from the break. Here's why: Electricity goes hand in hand with electromagnetic fields (EMFs). When something is plugged in but not used, it generates electrical fields, or low frequency electromagnetic waves. The EMFs create an invisible pollution called *electrosmog*.

Technology has gained a lot of traction over the last 50 years, spawning a multitude of new inventions that all require electricity. Everywhere you go you find electrical poles, wires, substations, transformers, and the hidden wires in the walls of every building. All this electricity creates a dangerous electrical environment and places new stresses on your cells similar to the ones produced by heavy metals or toxic chemicals.

You can't live in a bubble, but you can take some steps to reduce your exposure:

- ✔ **Remove yourself from the source as much as possible.** Make sure you aren't sleeping near a lot of wiring or electronic devices.

- ✔ **Eat foods that naturally shield your body.** Protect yourself against cellular damage by eating Paleo foods such as grass-fed beef, blueberries, asparagus, cinnamon, artichokes, garlic, olive oil, wild salmon, sea vegetables (nori), and walnuts. These choices are all superfoods for your cells.

- ✔ **Schedule a shut-down day.** Take one day per week and completely remove yourself from all electronics. Completely unplug.

If you want to test your house for EMF exposure, use a *gauss meter*. It's a small device (it fits in your pocket) that measures the strength of a magnetic field. You can pick one up for about $150 to $200. Use it to take measurements at home or work and see whether some areas are more exposed than others. You can see how far you need to be away from the TV or any electrical devices you choose.

Coming Together: Stress Management and the Paleo Lifestyle

If I had to pick one lifestyle factor that has had the biggest impact on my patients over the years, it'd definitely be their stress levels and ability to manage this stress.

What many people don't know is that stress not only makes you sick but also makes you fat. Society tends to equate weight problems with gorging on food, but the roots often go much deeper than that. Some people eat because they're hungry for something more in their life — like balance. Being under stress causes them to crave unhealthy foods without even realizing it.

This balance is one of the reasons that I love Paleo and that I believe it has so many raving fans. When you find food clarity and begin to dig into some of the recipes in Parts II through IV, your body starts normalizing. You create nutrient sufficiency and begin to regulate your hormones. You begin to gain the energy and the strength to deal with your stressors and create a better life.

This section digs a little deeper into how stress affects your body and your food choices, and I share some proven solutions for dealing with stress.

Examining your body under stress

Almost everything you do rises and falls on how much stress that activity places on your body. Some stress is short-term and can be positive (called *eustress*) if it gives you that short burst of adrenaline to move you closer to your purpose. For example, the stress of meeting deadlines to finish a book and share my nutritional message creates excitement and catalyzes me to move forward.

Your body isn't designed for constant, ongoing stress. Your stress hormones are in place to deal with short-term stress (such as being chased by a tiger). My body can handle the short-term stress of looming deadlines; however, if I kept pushing forward with an overwhelming schedule, the long-term stress would be adverse to my physiology and dangerous to my health. Balance really is the key.

Your body really does change under constant stress. Stress makes you heavy, makes your hair thin, ages your skin, and deteriorates all the structures and functions of your body. No wonder stress is a major contributor to illness, disease, and an unhappy life. So many diseases (such as heart disease, high blood pressure, and irritable bowel syndrome) stem from your body's having to deal with chronic stress.

Understanding how stress affects food choices

Here's information that can change your life: Sugar and fat are the main ingredients of stress hormones, so when you're under stress, you crave more sugar and fat than you do under normal conditions. That's when many people start stress eating to bring themselves down to a relaxed pace. In that way, *stress eating* is really a form of self-medication.

You're actually hard-wired to eat sugar and fat. Ideally, however, you'd follow your nutritional blueprint and get your fat and sugar from wild game, nuts, fruits, and vegetables like your ancestors did, not from all the refined sugary carbohydrates around today.

Ever notice when you crave sugar and fat the most? Dollars to donuts, it's when you're stressed. That's because of *serotonin* (or, rather, a lack of it). This hormone is a stress buffer; when your body is in balance, serotonin is released and offsets the activity in your body that leads to anxiety and depression. If you're constantly under stress, though, your body can't keep up with demand.

That's when you start feeling a mess. You eventually have increased stress hormones (such as *cortisol*) and decreased serotonin — a terrible combination. You become anxious, irritable, tired, and unhappy. You get changes in your appetite for — you guessed it — sugar and fat. It ends up being a vicious cycle that leads to even more stress.

Eating Paleo is a great way to step off the roller coaster. The fats that are part of the Paleo diet are all healthy fats, and the lower-sugar nature of the diet is really helpful in breaking negative eating patterns. For more tips on easing stress, check out the following section.

Finding stress solutions

When you bring your stress level down, you quell your cravings for sugar and fat. What I've found in listening to so many patients is that the answer to reducing stress is to have balance between work/stress and play/relaxation. So often, the people that come into my office seeking weight-loss management are heavy because their lives have gotten out of balance. They have too much stress and not enough tools to relax their bodies and bring them back to an even keel.

As I note throughout the chapter, living Paleo is about your choices. Ask yourself these questions before you make any decision: "Is this decision going to add a lot of stress in my life? Is it going to simplify my life or bring complexity to it?" Stress follows complexity. Learning to say "no" is one of the best stress-management tools you can develop!

Here are some suggested techniques to help you decompress. Make one of these options, or another healthy stress management technique you enjoy, part of your lifestyle:

- **Chiropractic:** Analyzes the body for nerve interference that occurs as a result of life's stresses. Many people feel immediately calmer after treatment. The later section "Improving your framework" has more info on incorporating chiropractic care into your life.

- **Massage:** Decreases the stress hormone cortisol and the hormones that can cause aggressive behavior.

- **Yoga and meditation:** Provide mental calmness, improved breathing, increased energy, and immunity.

- **The HeartMath Solution:** Calms the nervous system and creates positive mind body connections. Go to www.heartmath.org for more information.

✔ **Energy work:** Taps into that force within your body that gives you deep healing and strength. Chinese medicine, acupuncture, Qi Gong, Reiki, and Emotional Freedom Techniques (EFT) are just some of the techniques that center their healing on your body's life force (also called *prana, chi,* or *Qi*).

✔ **Exercise:** Boosts metabolism and changes the way your body responds to stress. Exercise is one of the most powerful things you can do to reverse stress, depression, anxiety, cravings, or negative eating patterns.

Probably the single most effective path to finding a practitioner or a technique that may be right for you is to ask a holistic practitioner (holistic MD, naturopath, or chiropractor) who knows your history about her recommendations. These folks are often very well connected to other practitioners in natural health and can recommend techniques and individual practitioners that suit your needs. If you don't know any such practitioners, just start asking around; people love to share this kind of information. Most of my patients have come to me by word of mouth. You can also find a Paleo practitioner at `http://paleophysiciansnetwork.com/doctors`.

Practicing Paleo Fitness: Movement by Design

If you could take a miracle pill every day that would decrease your incidence for about every disease, help you look better, moderate your cravings, and allow far less stress on your body, would you take it? Well, you already have this miracle pill; it's called exercise! Movement is a big part of living Paleo because it keeps your body healthy and makes all the structures and functions in your body work better. One of the best ways to stimulate your brain and hormones to produce pleasure is through exercise, so movement is great for elevating your mood as well. The following sections give you an overview of exercise's role in a Paleo lifestyle.

Paleo fitness covers so much more than I can address in a cookbook; check out my book with Melissa Joulwan, *Living Paleo For Dummies* (Wiley), for more background and an extensive workout schedule.

Making exercise a requirement, not an option

Exercise offers too many benefits for Paleo practitioners to ignore it. Your cells require exercise in order to be healthy; if you're deficient in anything that's required for healthy cell function, your overall health eventually suffers.

Here's the good news: Just as a deficiency in exercise can make you sick and obese, the reverse can work as well. You can use exercise to create healthy cells and robust health and even use it in place of some medications to heal your body and help fight aging.

Here are some of the medications that regular exercise may help you avoid:

- **Cold and flu meds:** The average adult has two or three colds or flu viruses each year. But if you're active, studies suggest that you'll have fewer colds than those who aren't.

- **Cholesterol meds:** Being active boosts your good cholesterol and reduces unhealthy triglycerides, keeping a clear pathway for blood to flow naturally and preventing conditions like diabetes, stroke, and heart disease.

- **Antidepressants:** If you work out three times per week hard enough to sweat, you can reduce depression just as well as an antidepressant can. The connections made between nerve cells while exercising behave as a natural antidepressant.

- **Respiratory/asthma meds:** When you exercise, your breathing becomes deeper, allowing more oxygen and nutrients to become more readily available.

- **Digestive aides:** Exercise stimulates your digestive juices, which creates movement through your bowels and helps prevent constipation.

- **Alzheimer's meds:** The *Archives of Neurology* published a report indicating that a daily walk or run may lower the risk of Alzheimer's disease or tame its impact.

- **Sedatives:** During exercise, your body releases chemicals called *endorphins.* These chemicals act as a sedative and create feelings of happiness and joy. Endorphins also decrease the perception of pain.

Keeping your modern-day body strong and lean

Existing in a world that you weren't designed for is certainly a challenge. Lifestyle patterns have moved away from what the human species requires to genetically express health and toward what causes it to express illness (sitting too much, sleeping too little, eating processed foods — the list goes on). How do you exist in this world and come out on the other end healthy, strong, and vibrant?

That's where living Paleo comes in. Your hunter-gatherer ancestors lived healthier lives. Regardless of what they died from, they were free from chronic illness and were healthy, fit, and full of vitality. They didn't have the maladies of modern civilization, such as heart attacks, strokes, diabetes, hypertension, and obesity. They were lean and strong.

The good news is you can mimic some of the lifestyle patterns of your ancestors and change the way you move by incorporating exercise into your everyday life.

Paleolithic peoples moved constantly and worked hard. Being physical was the center of their existence. If they wanted to eat, they had to work for it. If they wanted shelter, they had to work for it. They needed remarkable amounts of energy to provide their own clothing and even to prepare for bedtime. They were active and kept a vigorous pace.

That's where a big part of today's problems come in. With all the modern-day conveniences and affluence, people have gotten fat and lazy. In the Western world, people don't need to work for survival. Life in the wild may seem dangerous and unpredictable, but a modern-day sedentary life has just as many risks and uncertainties.

If you incorporate natural, functional movements like walking, crawling, sprinting, twisting, climbing, pushing, pulling, squatting, lifting, and throwing into your exercise routine, you train your body to use all of your muscles. This training helps you perform everything better (which is why these actions are often called *functional* movements). Whether you're chasing after kids or working as a professional athlete, a doctor, or an office worker, everything you do improves. Understanding natural movements is an important step in transforming your body into a lean, strong, modern-day physique.

High-intensity workouts that are shorter and faster get you strong and fit more quickly. This strategy allows your body to release growth hormone, which keeps you young. Your body puts on muscle, burns fat, and becomes metabolically conditioned. In fact, doing short bursts of exercise followed by rest is far better at getting you fit than all that long, stretched-out exercise that takes forever. That's got to be good news — that the exercise you need takes less time to be more effective! Short bursts of exercise not only give you fast results but also are way more practical for your busy life! Always think intensity, not time, when it comes to exercise.

Consider adding some high-intensity, natural movement into your routine two to three times per week, and watch your body transform into a leaner, stronger, younger, and healthier one!

Doing what you love

You need movement every day. About one hour should do it. That sounds like a lot, but remember, everything counts. Walking to your car, chasing after your kids, walking through the grocery store — it all matters.

Making time for about 20 minutes of high-intensity training two to three times per week is important for putting on muscle — which is one of the healthiest, most youth-promoting things you can do. The rest of the time, find movement you enjoy so you keep on keeping on! If you like to do yoga, hit the mat. If you like to hike, go for a hike. The idea is to just keep moving so that you get an hour a day.

Make sure that you exercise at a slower pace at least one day a week so you give your body the downtime it needs. Just because you may be moving at a slower pace doesn't mean it's not effective. This slower movement helps with daily stress, weight maintenance, blood sugar control, muscle tone, joint health, improved fat metabolism, a stronger immune system, and increased energy. As long as you're doing your high-intensity training and eating Paleo foods, you still benefit from slower movements.

Improving your framework

If you like to run, jump, push, pull, or lift anything, take care of your spine. It has one of the most important jobs of all the structures in your body: to protect your spinal column and allow you to bear weight. Your spine truly is the framework of your body; without it, you'd be like a jellyfish.

I've found that hands down, the most effective way to care for your spine is chiropractic care combined with exercise and spinal stretching. This combination is extraordinary for getting results. Many high-performers and high-profile people use chiropractic care as part of their best practices. My colleagues have adjusted music superstars, famous athletes, and countless other influential people who turn to chiropractic care because they know it helps them perform better.

Add chiropractic care and spinal stretching to your exercise routine for better posture and a healthier spine. You'll even notice improvements in your stress levels and immune system. To find a chiropractor in your area, go to www.findagreatchiro.com or http://paleophysiciansnetwork.com/doctors.

You can choose from many great spinal stretches that act like spinal floss to keep your spine healthy. Here's an all-time favorite of my patients called the Swiss ball stretch. If you have a large exercise ball like a Swiss ball, you can give your spine a nice stretch:

1. **Lie face up with the Swiss ball resting in the middle of your back and your feet planted on the floor.**

2. **Bring your arms up to a 90-degree angle at the shoulder and elbow.**

3. **Lean your head back and extend your spine as far back as you can go while keeping your feet planted on the floor, trying to touch your hands to the floor**

4. **Hold for 30 seconds.**

Check out this stretch in Figure 2-1. You won't want to get up! Just remember all your spine does for you and be sure you take the very best care of it.

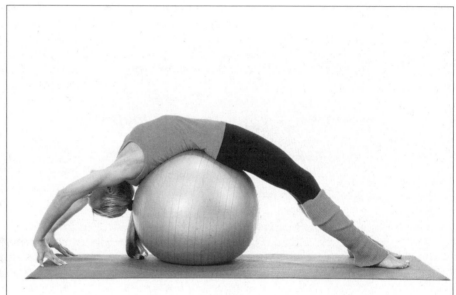

Figure 2-1: Swiss ball stretch.

Chapter 3

Discovering Paleo Superfoods

In This Chapter

▶ Introducing the Paleo superfoods

▶ Getting to know the Paleo yellow light foods

You've probably heard the term *superfood* tossed around before. So what's a superfood, exactly? It's food that's so nutrient dense and carries such nutritional excellence that it's the best raw material you can possibly give your cells. Bar none. *Paleo superfoods* are simply the healthiest foods on earth. They're the meat and eggs, fish and seafood, fruits, non-starchy and certain starchy vegetables, healthy fats and oils, and nuts and seeds that are in the optimal form for you to consume. If it's a Paleo superfood, it's got to be good!

When you get in the know about what these simple, natural foods are, going Paleo becomes second nature. The recipes in this book are all made with Paleo superfoods. As you go through the recipes and choose which ones you want to create, you begin to see how easy these superfoods are to use and enjoy. This chapter is your launch pad to discovering these foods.

Adopting a Paleo diet means the guesswork is over. That has to feel good — liberating, even. The framework of Paleo has set up a clear and definitive group of foods that are "yes" foods. You don't have to feel that food confusion you may have been dealing with in the past.

Green Light Foods: Loading Up on Paleo Superfoods

Paleo foods are by nature the real superfoods. Instead of thinking of Paleo as a diet, a way to heal conditions, or even a way to enhance athletic performance, think of it as simply eating the healthiest foods you can possibly consume.

That's it. Putting Paleo into the mixed bag of diets or healing remedies undersells and diminishes what it really is at the core. The Paleo-approved foods include the world's greatest superfoods, and they provide you with all the nutrition you'll ever need.

Your hunter-gatherer ancestors didn't have access to industrialized foods or planted crops, which means they didn't have grains, sugars, starches, legumes, dairy, or processed foods or oils. They survived on lean meats and eggs, fish and seafood, certain vegetables, certain fruits, nuts, seeds, and healthy fats — the same foods that make up the Paleo superfoods list in the following sections. Coincidence? I think not.

Meats, eggs, and bone broths

Protein builds and repairs you, increasing lean muscle mass and reducing body fat. Adequate protein supports your physique and ensures that your appetite is satisfied. The right quality protein supplies you with natural healthy fat.

- **Primal meats:** Wild animal meat — venison, rabbit, bear, and even wild boar — is an excellent protein choice. It's very lean and full of healthy omega-3 fatty acids.

- **Lean meats:** Your choices should always be free of antibiotics and other fillers. Beef, buffalo, lamb, goat, turkey, and chicken are all good sources. Just make sure your choices are always free of antibiotics and other fillers.

- **Organ meats:** Organ meats such as kidney, liver, and heart have a high concentration of fat-soluble vitamins; they're one of the best sources of vitamin D. They also have essential fatty acids. Be sure you get them from a healthy source to avoid toxins; I like U.S. Wellness Meats (www. grasslandbeef.com/StoreFront.bok).

- **Homemade bone broths:** *Bone broths* are flavorful liquids made from boiling animal bones for an extended period of time, often with vegetables or herbs, and then straining out the solids. The resulting broth is rich in vitamins, minerals, antioxidants, and amino acids. Bone broth is a powerful healer that reduces inflammation, heals infection, boosts immunity, stimulates bone health, heals the gut, and even has a calming effect. Check out the bone broth recipe in Chapter 18.

- **Eggs:** Rich in many key nutrients, especially fat-soluble vitamins A and D, egg yolk is also loaded with a B vitamin that's super brain food. Look for organic, pastured eggs with omega-3 for the best fatty acid profile.

If you choose to eat vegetarian protein sources, the most optimal choices are organic, non-GMO foods. (*GMO* refers to *genetically modified organisms,* which have had changes introduced into their DNA by genetic engineering techniques.) Avoid processed meatless burgers and so on. Instead, plant-based foods such as the following, which are closest to their natural state without all the processing, are your best choices:

- ✔ Tempeh
- ✔ *Natto* (steamed, fermented, and mashed soybeans)
- ✔ Edamame
- ✔ Beans
- ✔ High-quality protein powders, such as hemp or pea protein
- ✔ Full-fat yogurt and *kefir* (a fermented milk product) from milk of pasture-raised cows

Fish and seafood

Another valuable protein source to pile on your plate is wild-caught, sustainable fish. Your best bets are fattier, cold water fish such as salmon, sardines, mackerel, cod, and herring. Tuna packed in water is also a good choice. Be careful of fish packed in oil; the oil is often low-quality and rancid. If you eat seafood such as lobster, crab, shrimp, clams, or mussels, make sure you purchase from a reputable fishmonger who can tell you the source.

Your best tool for finding quality fish is to check out the Monterey Bay Aquarium Seafood Watch (`www.montereybayaquarium.org/cr/seafood watch.aspx`), which offers recommendations and a helpful mobile app.

Vegetables

Although protein is necessary to be super healthy, you can't just eat slabs of the proteins in the preceding sections and expect to be healthy. Balance is the key to building a healthy plate when it comes to the Paleo philosophy. You need to add some vegetables to your plate, too! Two different types of vegetables per meal are ideal.

These vegetables are Paleo superfoods because they harbor the most nutrition in them. They all have amazing healing, regenerating, and age-defying properties. Eating these vegetables help you boost immunity, perform better, and look and feel your best.

When your intentions exceed your budget

You may find yourself needing to purchase store-bought, conventional meat. Please don't stress about this. I always stress the importance of getting the best-quality meat you can, but you can still vastly improve your health just by cutting out many of the foods that your body isn't designed to have and including the ones that your body needs, like lean meats and eggs.

Buy the leanest cuts of red meat and poultry you can find, and drain the excess fat after cooking. Here are some better cuts of meat:

- Skinless chicken or turkey breast
- Eye of round roast or steak
- Sirloin tip side steak
- Top round roast and steak
- Bottom round roast and steak
- Top sirloin steak
- Lowfat ground beef

Here's the rundown of Paleo-approved superfood vegetables:

- **Cruciferous vegetables:** Cruciferous vegetables such as greens, kohlrabi, and the whole broccoli family, take the lead in the superfood vegetables category. They have sulfur-containing compounds that break down when you chew or chop them, causing a chemical reaction that boosts immunity.

- **Sea vegetables:** Sea vegetables are loaded with vitamins, minerals, antioxidants, and essential fatty acids. They nourish the thyroid, promote a healthy immune system, and prevent and treat many diseases. If you aren't familiar with sea veggies, here are some great choices:

  - Dulse

  - Hijiki

  - Kelp

  - Kombu

  - Nori

  - Wakame

- **Fermented vegetables:** Fermentation uses beneficial bacteria that are great for gut health. Because your gut health is so closely tied to your immunity and your skin health, fermented vegetables are a great superfood to add to your meals. Try kimchi or sauerkraut, or ferment some beets or carrots.

✔ **Miscellaneous vegetables:** Some vegetables, such as garlic, onions, spinach, and asparagus, are nutrient dense beyond what most vegetables can offer. They also have amazing healing and age-defying properties. Toss them in a salad, a soup, a stew, or even your morning eggs for a bit of a superfood blast!

Fruits

What I love about fruit is that it gives you the chance to sweeten things up a bit and still get nutrition. In fact, the darker the fruit's color, the more nutrition it usually contains. What really makes a fruit a superfood are the vitamins, minerals, disease-fighting phytochemicals, vision-promoting lutein, and fiber they contain. Some stand out from the pack:

✔ Apples

✔ Avocadoes

✔ Berries

✔ Cherries

✔ Grapefruit

✔ Kiwi

✔ Lemons

✔ Limes

✔ Mangoes

✔ Oranges

Nuts

Nuts and seeds are so popular because they taste great, are easily transportable, and carry a crunch. Unfortunately, these same characteristics make them easy to overdo.

Before you happily reach for the jar of nuts, note the catch: You need to consume these essential fats in the right ratios. The ideal fatty acid ratio should be about 4:1 omega-6 to omega-3. Unfortunately, the ratio of omega-6 to omega-3 in the modern diet is between 15:1 and 22:1. Most people are consuming far too much omega-6 fatty acid — about 15 to 20 times too much. Because nuts are slightly high on the omega-6 side, make sure you eat them in moderation only. The serving size is a closed handful (about ¼ cup).

These nuts stand out from the crowd for their healthier fatty acid profile, in addition to their low amount of polyunsaturated fats, which are unhealthy and can cause inflammation:

- Cashews
- Chestnuts
- Macadamia nuts
- Hazelnuts

Keep these nuts in the superfood category by buying the freshest available. You can ensure they are freshest when you buy the nut in the shell (never hulled). Always purchase raw nuts (except for cashews, which are unsafe eaten raw), buy in the bulk bins at the store where they move quickly, and store them in a cold dark place.

Fats and oils

Healthy fats make you look younger and help you lose weight; every structure and function in the body benefits from healthy oils.

You may think you're benefiting from an oil when you're actually consuming a damaged oil that's being cooked at too high a temperature. Overheating can damage some oils, causing oxidation that makes otherwise-healthy oils likely to cause inflammation. Avoid cooking with extra-virgin olive oil and nut oils; use those oils to toss on salads or drizzle over cooked food. For high-heat cooking — on the stovetop or grill or in the oven — use saturated fats from animals or coconut.

Superfood choices in the fats and oils category include the following:

- **Coconut fats:** Coconuts are an excellent source of saturated fat and produce so many delicious varieties of Paleo-approved fats: coconut oil (best for cooking), coconut butter, coconut flakes, and coconut milk.

- **Olives and avocadoes:** Both olives and avocadoes are favored sources of monounsaturated fats. Use olive oil and avocado oil for salads, and nibble on both olives and avocados in salads or as snacks.

- **Animal fats:** Animal fats are an excellent choice for cooking, but only if the fats come from organic, grass-fed, pastured animals. If you can find a good source, fats like lard, tallow, butter, and *ghee* (clarified butter) are healthful, delicious options.

Coconut-based pantry foods

The pantry foods that stand out from the crowd are the fabulous coconut products. Coconut is a magnificent antibacterial and antimicrobial food. It promotes weight loss, a healthy immune system, and a healthy metabolism; keeps your skin healthy and youthful-looking; and is one of the best oils you can cook with because it stays stable at such high temperatures.

- ✔ Coconut aminos (an alternative to soy)
- ✔ Coconut butter
- ✔ Unsweetened coconut flakes
- ✔ Canned coconut milk
- ✔ Coconut oil

Always double-check the label on pantry items just to be extra sure you aren't getting any nasty ingredient surprises.

Yellow Light: Approaching Some Foods with Caution

Some foods may fall into a bit of a gray area for Paleo aficionados. When your body is healthy and your gut is strong, you may make some food decisions that fall outside of the realm of strict Paleo. The following sections help you navigate those fuzzy areas while choosing the best, most superfood options available.

Doing dairy

Some people can handle dairy, and others can't. Personally, I can't touch it; it has almost an immediate reaction on my body. I can tolerate some grass-fed butter and ghee, but that's where it ends with me.

However, if you're one of those folks who feel like dairy is no issue with you, get only the highest-quality full-fat dairy and tune in to how dairy affects your body. Be sure you aren't experiencing any symptoms of dairy intolerance, such as earaches, acne, congestion, joint aches, yeast infections, premenstrual discomfort, fatigue, asthma, skin rashes, or intestinal issues.

When you eat the "gold standard" dairy products — raw, fermented, full-fat dairy such as cultured butter, yogurt, kefir, and cheese — you're getting a healthy fat, a fermented food, and *conjugated linoleic acid,* which has tremendous healing affects.

Making superfood produce work with intestinal issues

Raw foods are full of vitamins and make you super healthy. In fact, I love them so much I think it's a benefit to have some raw produce with every meal. However, when raw fruits and veggies become an intestinal irritant, they're no longer in your best interest to eat. You may have to just give your body a break for awhile until it heals. The great news is that when you eat Paleo foods, you're doing all you can to get as healthy as possible.

If you have minor intestinal issues (such as bloating, discomfort, and gas) or more-serious conditions (such as irritable bowel syndrome [IBS], Crohn's disease, colitis or ulcerative colitis, or celiac disease), you may want to pull back on the raw foods, cooking your vegetables thoroughly until you heal. Here are some ways to get your superfood produce during this time:

- **Predigest.** Predigest your vegetables as much as possible by chopping them into small pieces and chewing them thoroughly.

- **Slow cook.** For low-grade intestinal issues, slow cooking vegetables in dishes such as soups or stews makes them easier to digest.

- **Limit fruit.** Eat small quantities of fruit until your body has fully transitioned into its healing phase. Stay away from dried fruit for a few months until your intestines have the digestive strength. If you have one of the more-serious intestinal conditions, avoid any fruit you can't peel until the healing phase gains traction; that exterior of the fruit may be too much roughage for your body to handle.

- **Don't drink and eat.** If you have intestinal disorders, hold off on drinking while you eat. Instead, wait until 20 minutes after finishing before you take a swig. This strategy keeps your digestive juices from getting diluted; they stay as strong as possible so they can work at breaking your food down as fully as possible. The more they break raw foods down, the less likely those foods are to irritate your intestinal lining.

Maybe foods

Maybe foods aren't technically Paleo foods, but you may feel like they're okay to have once in a while. In these instances, savor the experience and enjoy every bite.

For example, if you're going to France and want to indulge in a croissant, make sure you hold out for the real deal; don't chow down on the first imitation pastry you're offered on the flight over. If you're going out for sushi, make sure it's not just the grocery store pick-up version. The same applies to special occasions. Just pull back to the Paleo superfoods when you know you need to.

Warning: These maybe foods guidelines don't apply to those with bowel disorders such as irritable bowel syndrome (IBS), Crohn's disease, colitis, ulcerative colitis, or celiac disease. If you have one of these conditions, adhere as absolutely closely as possible to your Paleo superfoods.

Alcohol

Although no alcoholic beverages are superfoods, some are definitely better than others. When you want the occasional happy hour beverage, these Paleo drinks fit the bill because they don't have gluten:

- ✔ Organic red wine
- ✔ Organic white wine
- ✔ Organic sparkling wine
- ✔ Potato vodka
- ✔ Tequila
- ✔ Rum

 Choose drier wines, which have less sugar. Pinot Noir, Cabernet Sauvignon, and Merlot are good red choices; for white wines, try Sauvignon Blanc and Albariño.

 If you have a digestive disorder of some type, you should avoid alcohol 100 percent of the time because it can further damage your gut.

Chapter 4

Launching the 30-Day Reset

*T*his chapter is about resetting your body so it functions at a higher level. When your body recalibrates, you start naturally losing fat, your eyes brighten, and your skin glows. You begin to think more clearly, and your mood lifts. All these benefits are yours when you create a healthy environment and provide your body with deep, sufficient nutrition.

Just think of it this way: Where there is waste, there is weight. Where there is deficiency, there is illness. The Paleo Reset is your answer to all these situations. Your body fine-tunes and refines to a healthier state.

When your body isn't working hard to deal with what it doesn't need, it focuses on getting you more of what you do need. You get healthier, stronger, and leaner. When you take the time to clear out your body's waste, you'll be shocked how your body composition begins to change and your energy skyrockets.

The best way to transition to a Paleo lifestyle and diet is with a 30-Day Reset. In this chapter, I explain the Reset and its benefits beyond simply getting you on the Paleo track. I also highlight specific foods and portions that are appropriate during the 30-Day Reset, and I answer some of the most commonly asked questions regarding the Reset and how it will work for you.

What's a Paleo Reset Anyway?

A *Paleo Reset* is a way of eating for 30 days that creates the healthiest possible environment in your body for you to have long-term success with living Paleo. The Reset helps you achieve all the positive benefits of a Paleo lifestyle like losing weight, boosting immunity, healing conditions, and feeling energized and youthful. A Paleo Reset isn't a powder, a liquid, or pills you take hoping to clean out your system.

The fluid around your cells is your *internal milieu,* and this fluid must be healthy for you to be healthy. Think of your body like a fish tank. The water in your tank is your internal milieu. When you eat healthy and balanced food, you nourish this milieu; when you eat poorly, you clog and acidify this system, your cells become like sludge, and you look and feel toxic — like fish trying to survive in a dirty tank. The Paleo Reset helps clean out your fish tank and gives you a clean, fresh start.

I know the Paleo Reset seems intimidating. I know it seems strict and even hard. But remember what's truly hard: healing your body of serious disease or going through the depression of knowing that you're not living your life because you're tired, in pain, or overweight. From this perspective, 30 days is just a drop in the bucket. The Reset is challenging, and it's going to take some grit, but it's well worth the effort to get from where you are now to where you want to be.

Reaping the benefits of the Reset

When you commit to the 30-Day Reset, you jump-start your body's improvement in every way. Your body begins

- **Eliminating toxins:** When you drink plenty of water, toxins leave through liver, lungs, intestines, and kidneys.

- **Slaying your sugar cravings:** You're breaking sugar addiction, and your body is switching to using fat for fuel rather than using sugar and sugary carbohydrates.

- **Getting your gut health in order:** Every 21 days, your intestinal cells turn over (regenerate). All the *nutrient dense* foods (foods with lots of nutrients compared to their calories) you feed your body during the Reset provide the best raw material to form the healthiest cells possible.

- **Reducing inflammation:** The healthy fats and clean foods of the Reset quiet inflammation throughout your entire body. This concept is one of the cornerstones of eating Paleo.

- **Rebuilding and healing:** All the structures and functions of your body begin to strengthen.

- **Balancing your fatty acids:** Your ratio of omega-6 to omega-3 fatty acids improves, which is great for reducing inflammation.

✔ **Optimizing your metabolism:** The balance of *macronutrients* (the protein, carbohydrates, and fat that provide you with energy) helps you create an efficient metabolism.

✔ **Balancing blood sugar:** The foods on the Paleo Reset help stabilize your blood sugar for the long term.

In addition, during the 30-Day Reset you begin to break unhealthy food habits. How much you eat, what you choose to eat, and the pleasure you connect with food are often the end results of a habit you've created. You may not even realize that what you're doing isn't healthy or getting you to where you want to be. These 30 days begin to address these concerns and reprogram your habits.

When you regulate your body signals with healthy Paleo foods, you learn to just let your body decide naturally when it needs to eat. Your body gets into a natural rhythm, and you can more easily determine when your body really is hungry. Letting your body tell you when it needs to eat is much more efficient than forcing yourself to eat just because it's supposed to be mealtime.

You also create an awareness of your food that you've never had before. You begin to pay attention to high-nutrient foods and to notice how many packaged foods you've been eating. Best of all, you become aware of how certain foods make you feel, which is paramount for long-term success. These cues are what help you understand which foods agree with your system and which ones don't.

Think about it: If you can invest 30 days in something that will make an impact for the rest of your life, isn't it worth a try?

Putting real foods first

The most important concept of the Paleo Reset is simply about making sure that all the foods you choose are from real food sources, with a focus on quality. You don't put anything with a bar code past your lips for 30 days. That's it. You don't need any special pills or juices.

Trying to explain this concept to patients who are so eager to walk out the door with a "bottle of something" to cleanse is always interesting. It's kind of like the Abbott and Costello skit "Who's On First?":

Patient: "Doc, I really think I need a cleanse."

Me: "I agree; let's get you started. I'm going to ask you to eat nothing with a bar code for 30 days."

Patient: "Okay, what do I take?"

Me: "You don't need to take anything. Let's just start by having you eat nothing with a bar code for 30 days."

Patient: "Okay, but don't I need something to cleanse me?"

Me: "The foods will cleanse you."

Patient: "Oh, good. So what supplements do I need to buy to get started?"

Me: "Nothing. You're good to go. We'll go over your food plan and what to expect for the next 30 days, and you'll be set."

Patient: "Okay, but what do I take to actually *cleanse?*"

Me: [sigh]

During the 30-Day Reset, you eat super clean with whole foods, without any of the Paleo-friendly treats (such as grain-free muffins, pancakes, or desserts) that are okay after the Reset. You focus on eating quality meats, fish, and eggs; healthy fats; Paleo-approved vegetables and fruits; and nuts and seeds.

The three most essential points over the 30 days are to keep your foods simple, balanced, and of the highest quality you can afford. You concentrate on the foods you're designed to eat and that give your body what it craves to be strong, lean, and healthy.

After you do the 30 days, you quickly realize that foods with deep nutrition are your launching pad to a life of looking and feeling amazing. Your food choices and your relationship with food change after you experience the 30-Day Reset.

Understanding why you need 30 days

You've likely spent a long time developing your eating habits, so breaking them and instituting new ones may take some time. The longer you've depended on sugary foods, the more difficult retraining your taste buds to recognize natural sweetness may be.

The Reset lasts 30 days for three reasons:

- ✔ **Allowing time for cell regeneration:** All your organs regenerate themselves constantly. Your body's motive is to get rid of all the weak, sick cells and replace them with healthy cells. Your cells have different life spans, and your intestinal cells take about 21 days to renew. That's why starting your Paleo program with a 30-Day Reset is important: 30 days gives you enough time to encompass a full intestinal regeneration cycle, so you start out your new lifestyle with healthy, vibrant cells.

✔ **Creating positive habits:** Your nervous system takes about 30 days to recognize a habit. When you do something over and over for about 30 days, you start getting the hang of it and moving in the right direction. Your actions may not be completely automatic yet and may take some forethought, but chances are that within 30 days, you're reaching for that crinkly package a lot less frequently.

✔ **Quieting the cravings:** What's really behind your cravings? Sometimes, your body is looking for ways to find comfort. The brain chemical that's responsible for this reaction is called *serotonin;* it affects mood — specifically, happiness. The higher your serotonin levels, the happier you feel. When these levels dip, you may turn to sweets or processed foods as an artificial way to elevate these levels.

Doing the 30 day Paleo Reset forces you to find ways to naturally increase this feel-good guy serotonin. Exercising, thinking positive thoughts, and eating the clean, nutritious Paleo foods are some of the best ways to naturally boost these serotonin levels and win this epic battle once and for all.

The difference between the first 30 days and simply eating Paleo for life is that a long-term Paleo lifestyle gives you a bit of wiggle room in your food choices — what I like to call *personal play.* The 30-Day Reset, though, has no room for these different shades of Paleo. You avoid the Paleo-approved sweets and treats; (such as pancakes, muffins, and sugars of any kind) that are okay later; straight-up, 100-percent squeaky-clean Paleo foods are the only focus during this period. You have to be strict with your portion sizes as well. No cheating or swaying, or it's back to day number one!

Earning willpower

You may be considering a Paleo Reset and thinking, "But I don't have any willpower." No one *has* willpower. Willpower is something that's developed. Just like building muscles, you must build your physiology to have willpower to become mentally fit.

Every time you exercise self-control, you're strengthening your willpower. So when you see that person happily eating spaghetti squash and you want to cry into a bowl of real pasta, it doesn't mean that she has more willpower than you; it just means she has more mental conditioning and has practiced more self-control in her life. (Or maybe she just flat-out likes spaghetti squash more than you do). It's a numbers game, really. The more you exercise willpower, the easier it becomes.

You can actually work on willpower by holding back on doing something you really want to do When you push your mental muscle beyond its limits, you eventually cause it to tire, but like your bicep, when you exercise to exhaustion you actually cause your mental muscle to strengthen.

After 30 days, when you've reduced inflammation, worked on healing your gut, stabilized your blood sugar, and become a more efficient fat burner, you can venture out beyond the 30-Day Reset menu. Most of my patients experience the best results when they stick to a diet that's 80 percent Paleo and 20 percent personal play.

Some folks need more than 30 days before they are ready to have flexibility. If you have a condition you are trying to heal, you may decide to continue on past the 30 days. Again, what works for you personally is an important part of eating Paleo.

Feeling shaky, crazy, and tired

Be aware of what's happening when you launch the 30-Day Reset. If you start to feel a bit wonky as you're switching over your diet to Paleo foods, know that you're A-Okay. This yucky feeling is actually a signal that your body is making a positive switch. Some folks feel mental fuzziness, headaches, fatigue, achy joints, or shakiness during some part of their first 30 days. Think of this discomfort as an accomplishment because your body is actually conquering carbs. That's why this time is often called the *carb flu*. Your body is making the nasty transition from burning carbohydrates for energy to burning fats for energy. Just try to be patient; on average, it takes four to seven days to get through the carb flu, but for some it may take longer. Just hang tight and know that this side effect is just part of your transition.

Here's what's happening during this process physically: Your body needs glucose (sugar) for the brain, muscles, cells, and so on to function. Before you started eating Paleo, glucose was easy to access from all the sugary carbohydrates you were likely eating. Now, without the constant carb supply, your body has to create some of the glucose it needs from fats and proteins, which isn't an easy process.

So What Can I Eat? Recognizing Your 30-Day Reset Power Foods

During the 30-Day Reset, you concentrate on providing the best raw material to rebuild a strong, healthy body: lean meats, fish and eggs, healthy fats, Paleo approved vegetables, fruits, and nuts and seeds (see Figure 4-1). These simple, real foods help you get back to the basics. The essential point is that you should keep your foods simple, balanced, and of the highest quality your budget allows.

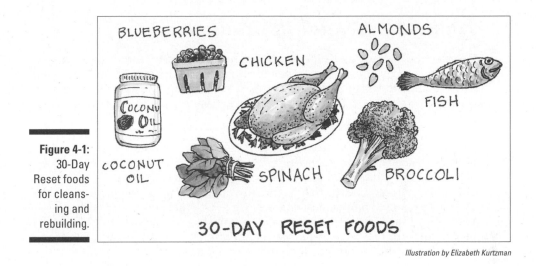

BLUEBERRIES ALMONDS

CHICKEN

COCONUT OIL

FISH

COCONUT OIL

SPINACH BROCCOLI

30-DAY RESET FOODS

Figure 4-1: 30-Day Reset foods for cleansing and rebuilding.

Illustration by Elizabeth Kurtzman

Picking the right Reset proteins

Purchasing your meat and eggs from pasture-raised, organic sources and seafood from a sustainable, wild source is the ideal (both during the Reset and in general). The guidelines for choosing proteins for the Reset are the same as the ones for everyday Paleo; check out Chapters 5 and 6 for more details on buying the following proteins:

- ✔ **Eggs and egg whites**
- ✔ **Poultry**
- ✔ **Beef**
- ✔ **Lamb**
- ✔ **Wild game**
- ✔ **Canned fish (tuna, salmon, sardines, mackerel)**
- ✔ **Pork/boar products**
- ✔ **Deli meats and chicken or turkey sausage**
- ✔ **Fish, seafood, and shellfish**

If you're on a strict budget, meat is where I recommend you shell out the extra bucks. Healthy meat is more difficult to find on a budget than other healthy Paleo-approved conventional foods are. If your grocery budget doesn't allow you to invest in higher-quality protein right now, that's okay. If you must buy conventionally raised meat, you can find tips to help improve its healthfulness in Chapter 5.

Focusing on quality produce

Because the 30-Day Reset's focus is on balance, simplicity, and quality, choose fruits and veggies that are in season for the freshest, most nutritious options. And if your favorite isn't available fresh, frozen fruits and vegetables — because they're flash-frozen in season just after picking — are a solid, nutritious alternative to fresh.

Non-starchy vegetables are yours for the taking. Try new and interesting vegetables to keep it exciting. The best rule of thumb when you think vegetables is to think rainbow. Get as many different vegetables in as many different colors as you can. These bright colors are an indication of the phytonutrients the foods contain; more color means more good stuff. Focus your starchy vegetable intake (sweet potatoes, winter squash, and other roots and tubers) in the post-workout eating window to minimize their blood-sugar-raising effect. Try kohlrabi or jicama for a new and different starchy vegetable.

All fresh Paleo-approved fruit is okay during the Reset, but my favorite choices during the 30 days are those that have a minimum impact on blood sugar and add great flavor: lemons, limes, berries, avocadoes, apples, and grapefruit. Avoid fruit juices, sweetened fruits, and dried fruits during the Reset to avoid blood sugar swings.

Eat no more than two servings of fruit per day. Break those servings up across meals and snacks to distribute your sugar intake and release less insulin. The later section "Sizing Up Reset-Friendly Portions" has details on appropriate serving sizes.

The Environmental Working Group (EWG; www.ewg.org/foodnews/) did testing on produce and found which types are most beneficial to buy organic because of high pesticide contamination. You can find the EWG shopping list recommendations in Chapter 5.

Seeking Reset spices

Spices are an especially nice addition during your 30-Day Reset because of the additional healing they may provide. During this time, your body is focusing on healing and regulating. Spices such as cinnamon, ginger, and turmeric can help heal your body as well as provide flavor. For more information on spices, head to Chapter 5.

Fixating on Reset-friendly fats

All Paleo-approved fats are approved for the Reset, including the following (see Chapter 5 for more details):

- ✔ **Coconut fats**

- ✔ **Olives and avocadoes**

- ✔ **Animal fats**

- ✔ **Nuts, seeds, nut and seed oils, and nut and seed butters**

Cooking at high heat can damage some oils, causing oxidation that makes otherwise-healthy oils likely to cause inflammation. Avoid cooking with extra-virgin olive oil and nut oils; instead, use those oils to toss on salads or drizzle over cooked food. For high-heat cooking — on the stovetop or grill or in the oven — use saturated fats from animals or coconut-sourced fats.

- ✔ **High-heat oils:** Coconut oil, palm oil, ghee (clarified butter), and animal fats

- ✔ **Low-heat oils:** Macadamia nut oil and avocado oil

- ✔ **No-heat oils (cold use only):** Olive oil, walnut oil

These oils are so bad, they don't even belong in a landfill. Keep these out of your house during your Reset and beyond:

- ✔ Canola oil (rapeseed oil)

- ✔ Cottonseed oil

- ✔ Grapeseed oil

- ✔ Margarine

- ✔ Partially hydrogenated vegetable oil

- ✔ Rice bran oil

- ✔ Safflower oil

- ✔ Soybean oil

- ✔ Sunflower oil

- ✔ Vegetable oil and shortening

Sipping on Reset beverages

Drink pure, natural beverages, and stay away from anything that's going to spike your blood sugar. Chapter 5 has a list of Paleo-approved beverages, all of which are acceptable for the Reset.

During these 30 days, make sure you have no sweetener whatsoever, including stevia, honey, maple syrup, agave, and even coconut palm sugar.

Packing the pantry for your Reset

Although the main focus of the 30-Day Reset is basic nuts-and-bolts foods, you can explore a bit into some Reset-ready pantry foods. Here's the rundown:

- Beef and chicken broth (I recommend Imagine brand)
- Canned chilies
- Canned fish (watch the label for soy, sugar, or other unhealthy ingredients)
- Canned coconut milk
- Canned vegetables (sweet potatoes, squash, and pumpkin)
- Clarified butter or ghee (I recommend Pure Indian Foods brand)
- Coconut aminos
- Coconut butter
- Coconut flakes (unsweetened)
- Coconut oil
- Curry paste (I recommend Thai Kitchen brand)
- Fish sauce (I recommend Red Boat brand)
- Hot sauce
- Jerky (I recommend Primal Pacs or Gourmet Grassfed brands)
- Mustard (watch the label for sugar, cornstarch, maltodextrin, or other unhealthy ingredients)
- Olives (watch the label for sulfites)
- Pickles and relish
- Salsa
- Sun-dried tomatoes
- Tomato sauce and paste
- Vinegar, all varieties except malt
- 100 percent unsweetened cocoa powder

Sizing Up Reset-Friendly Portions

Three variables determine how much you eat every day:

- ✔ Your hunger level
- ✔ Your energy level
- ✔ Your exercise/activity level

Most people aren't aware of how much they eat in a day. During the 30-Day Reset, pay attention to portion sizes. After that, recognizing correct portions becomes second nature; you automatically know how much should be on your plate. For the 30-Day Reset, here's a basic template of serving sizes:

- ✔ **Protein:** Each meal should include a serving of protein. A serving of meat, fish, or poultry should be about the size and thickness of your palm (see Figure 4-2). That's about 3 to 4 ounces for women and 5 to 6 ounces for men. A serving of eggs is as many eggs as you can easily hold in your hand. That's about two or three for women and three or four for men. To gauge a serving of egg whites, double the number of whole eggs. (Remember, though that the yolk contains good stuff: B vitamins, zinc, and *choline,* which transports cholesterol through your body.)

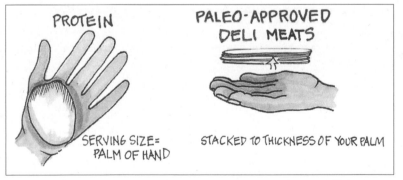

Figure 4-2:
Protein
serving size.

Illustration by Elizabeth Kurtzman

- ✔ **Non-starchy vegetables:** A serving of non-starchy vegetables should be at least the size of a softball. Fill your plate with at least two or three softballs' worth — whatever the amount you need to reach satiety. When it comes to these veggies, you can't eat too many!

- ✔ **Starchy vegetables:** *Starchy vegetables* are your more carbohydrate-dense options such as sweet potato, jicama, kohlrabi, or squash. A serving of starchy vegetables should be about 1 cup for women and 1½ cups for men.

✔ **Fruit:** A serving of fruit is half an individual piece (for example, half an apple or half an orange) or a tennis-ball-size serving of berries, grapes, or tropical fruits. That's a closed fistful if they're diced — about half a cup.

✔ **Liquid fats:** A serving of liquid fat should be about the size of a ping-pong ball or your thumb. That's about 1 tablespoon. Each meal should include one to two servings of fat (see Figure 4-3).

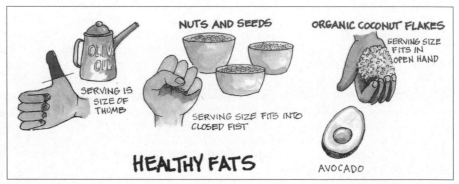

Figure 4-3:
Fat serving size.

Illustration by Elizabeth Kurtzman

✔ **Nuts and seeds:** A serving is about one closed handful.

✔ **Coconut flakes and olives:** A serving fits into your open hand (see Figure 4-3).

✔ **Avocado:** A serving is one-quarter to one-half of the avocado as shown in Figure 4-3.

✔ **Coconut milk:** A serving is one-third to one-half of the can.

Keep in mind that you have some personal wiggle room with these serving guidelines. If you find yourself hungry all the time, make adjustments and eat more!

Some people do great on three meals and allow their body the break in between meals to burn fat for fuel. Others need a snack to get them through the morning or afternoon. Paleo is flexible enough to support whatever your body needs. Your snacks should be about half the size of your meals and should always include protein and healthy fat. Paleo-approved fat in particular really helps curb cravings during the 30-Day Reset. Here are some great Reset snack options:

✔ Almonds or almond butter with an apple or celery

✔ Coconut butter

✔ Handful of unsweetened coconut chips

✔ Mashed avocado or guacamole with sliced veggies

✔ Paleo-approved jerky

✔ Paleo-approved turkey lunchmeat rolled up with avocado and mustard

✔ Smoked salmon wrapped in nori sheets

Addressing Common Questions about the 30-Day Reset

You decided to commit and go for the 30-Day Reset. Fantastic! But what about those nagging questions? How do you get away from feeling lost, aimless, or like a weirdo? Easy! In this section, I tackle what I call the big hitter questions that I get in my practice, at dinner parties, on the running trail, at the dentist, at the mall — you get my drift. Any question you have, I probably cover it here! And if you've dug up a question I haven't touched on, tweet me your question: @drkellyann. I'll get you an answer!

These 30 days are about you! Whatever adjustments you have to make in your crazy, awesome life will be well worth their (unprocessed) salt to get these 30 days done. This 30-Day Reset is the best cleanse you could ever give your body and mind. You'll see — and so will everyone else!

✔ **Can I put salt on my food?** Well, salt can either kill ya or make ya well. Quality matters here in a big way. If you eat table salt, you're eating a refined food. If you eat a pure, natural salt, you're eating minerals that support you. I've used Celtic sea salt for years and find it to be really pure and filled with minerals.

When you do make the switch to a high-quality salt, you don't get iodine from it because iodine isn't naturally occurring in salt. To counteract this problem, incorporate some of the following Reset-friendly iodine sources:

- Seaweed such as kelp, nori, and dulse

- Proteins such as eggs, meat, and poultry

- Vegetables such as Swiss chard, asparagus, and spinach

- Strawberries

My favorite way to get iodine is to mash some nori sheets in soup or a salad or use them as a wrap.

✔ **What kind of sweetener can I use?** You may not like this one, but for 30 days, the answer is "nothing." Just get this done, and your sugar cravings will really diminish.

✔ **Can I have alcohol? I really like wine at night.** For 30 days, alcohol in all forms (even for cooking) is a no-go. All those things I promise you about healing your gut, building better cells, cutting sugar cravings, boosting your immunity, and so on aren't going to happen if you're drinking alcohol. Can you white knuckle this one for 30 days? You'll be glad you did.

✔ **Can I take vitamins?** Yes. However, you're flooding your body with so many nutrients that you probably won't need much in the way of out-side supplementation other than fish oil, vitamin D, and for some, a pro-biotic if some extra healing power is needed.

✔ **Are nut butters okay?** Yes! In moderation, all nut butters (except for peanut butter) are okay. Many people find it reassuring to know that sunflower seed butter (found in most grocery stores) is even a good replacement for peanut butter. The serving size for these items is two tablespoons. Check the labels to make sure you're not getting stuff you don't want, such as added sugar.

✔ **I love butter on my sweet potatoes. Can I use it just for that?** Nope, sorry. I know, I know. It seems ridiculous that you can't have a little butter on a sweet potato, but no dairy means no dairy. However, ghee and clarified butter are okay because the sugars, water, and milk solids (including the often troublesome lactose and casein) have been removed. Just make sure your butter is from a grass-fed source so you're getting the full nutritional value.

✔ **What in the world can I eat for breakfast?** If I had a penny for every time a patient asked me what to have for breakfast, I'd be writing this book from my private island. I know eggs get old, but eggs are just a super healthy protein that fuels your brain and body. If you can't bear the thought of one more morning with eggs, here's another idea: Whatever protein you cook at night, make some extra for your breakfast. As I note in Chapter 11, breakfast doesn't have to center on traditional breakfast foods.

One of my favorite breakfasts is salmon and a handful of berries. Another is protein with some kimchi. Keep an avocado around for a great breakfast fat because it's so versatile, or just grab some coconut flakes or a teaspoon of coconut butter with a protein. Even a nut butter right out of the jar works.

✔ **How much are these 30 days going to cost me?** The truth is, I can't tell you buying superior-quality foods that can change and possibly save your life costs less than buying a breakfast muffin at the quick mart. I can tell you this much though — most people have no idea how much they're eating. Prepare to be amazed when you find out how little food your body really needs to be satisfied when eating foods with a high nutritional density. You may actually end up spending less on food over-all because you're buying fewer packaged foods! You may have some initial cost layout when you stock up, but in the long run, you can seek out deals through farm markets, big box stores, and store sales. I know many families who eat 100-percent Paleo foods on very little means.

✔ **I feel like I can't eat anything. Am I getting the nutrients I need?** Let me clear up the idea of missing nutrients once and for all:

- **Fiber:** You get plenty of fiber from fruits and vegetables, which are much more digestible sources than grains or beans are.

- **Calcium:** Plant sources such as kale, spinach, and collard greens as well as other sources such as shrimp, salmon, and olives provide you with loads of calcium — without the inflammation dairy brings for so many people.

- **Vitamins and minerals:** Real food equals real nutrition, and what better way to get immune-building nutrients than with lean proteins, healthy fats, vegetables, and fruit? You're definitely covered! You don't need grains, dairy, legumes, or soy when you have nutrient dense foods like the Paleo foods.

✔ **But I have my friend's wedding coming up, and I go out to dinner a lot. What happens if I screw up?** Unfortunately, slip-ups mean going back to day 1. If you stop and start, the inflammation isn't going to leave and you're not going to figure out your intolerances or reset your cells. If you want results, you have to do 30 consistent days. That said, rest assured that you'll discover how to get around these situations. Eating protein and vegetables isn't hard — no matter where you go. I carry my own sea salt and oil just about everywhere.

✔ **I'm really hungry. Am I supposed to be hungry?** Often, being hungry is your body's way of recalibrating to a new system. You've removed all the carbohydrate-dense, nutrition-poor foods such as packaged, processed, sugary carbs, grains, and legumes that may have been the source of most of your calories. Replacing these calories with healthy fats from grass-fed animal fats, coconut, or avocado plus quality proteins and vegetables fuels your body efficiently and sustains you so your hunger diminishes with healthy raw material.

Be sure to drink enough water. Your body can often confuse the thirst signal as a hunger signal. A general rule is to drink about half your body weight in ounces of water throughout the day. Also make sure you're getting enough protein and fat, which can help sustain you.

✔ **I'm a vegetarian. Can I do the Reset?** If your brand of vegetarianism allows you to eat some eggs and fish, being a Paleo vegetarian is pretty simple. Just try to build your plate with those foods as your protein and use the plant-based proteins (such as *tempeh* [fermented cooked soybean], beans, or tofu) only as the exception, not the rule. Eating plenty of eggs and fish along with veggies, fruits, and nuts ensures you get the protein you need.

On the other hand, if you choose not to eat any meat, fish, or eggs, you have to look to other vegetarian protein to get your nutrition. The best choices for following a vegetarian Paleo diet are organic, dense protein sources, like non-GMO plant-based foods, including the following:

- Tempeh

- *Natto* (steamed, fermented, and mashed soybeans)

- Edamame

- Tofu

- Beans: Lentils, black beans, pinto beans, and red beans

- High-quality protein powders, hemp, or pea protein

- Full-fat, pasture-raised yogurt and *kefir* (a fermented milk product) if dairy isn't an issue for you

These aren't the most optimal foods in general because many of them are mucus forming and cause inflammation. But you do need to get protein somewhere, so if you can't fathom eating any kind of meat, these are your best bets. Just be sure you're getting vitamin B12 and eating Paleo approved healthy fats to reduce any inflammation. (I recommend seeing your health practitioner to get your B12 level checked as a baseline; many vegetarians tend to run a bit low on B12. If you are a vegetarian and need a non-food source of this vitamin, B12 shots tend to have the best absorption.)

Some protein options just aren't healthy for anyone. Period. In fact, the following options aren't even foods. They're *food products* — what I like to call *frankenfoods* — and are usually a mixture of a wheat protein with a subpar oil.

- Soy milk
- Tofu hot dogs
- Veggie bacon
- Veggie chicken
- Veggie chicken wings
- Veggie loafs
- Veggie "sausage" links

Responding to doubters and naysayers

"People think I'm crazy for eating this way. What do I tell them?" It stupefies me that people think it's "weird" that your diet consists of real foods. Yet processed, denatured frankenfoods made up of scary, unpronounceable stuff are the norm, so you'll probably have to deal with someone in your life questioning your food choices.

Nothing can make you feel more deflated than when you start getting in the swing of living Paleo and are ambushed with negativity about being on some "strange diet kick." The best way to diffuse all the pressure surrounding the issue of your food choices is to remain positive, smile when approached, and most importantly, be grounded in why you're doing what you're doing. You're not going to carry any influence whatsoever if you get preachy, frustrated, or annoyed at people coming head to head with you.

Living Paleo is a new paradigm for a lot of people, and adjusting to this mindset takes time. Holding back when you're really excited about something is tough, I know. But let people come to you when they're ready. The best thing you can do is provide people with your walking testimonial of transformation. When you start looking and feeling your best, don't be surprised if the same people razzing you are the same people that come up to you and say, "How do I start with this Paleo thing?" You can practically set your watch to it. Let your improved lab results or athletic performance, changed appearance, and your renewed energy be the topic of discussion. Talk about the amazing foods you get to eat and how Paleo cooking has gotten you back in the kitchen.

Remember: Tread very lightly when backing up your food choices to others by citing "the science behind Paleo." You had better know your stuff like nobody's business because someone is bound to pull out a counterargument based on her view on science, and, well, these discussions can get ugly.

I love the "Nutrition in 60 Seconds" pitch that Dallas and Melissa Hartwig of http://whole9life.com came up with in their book *It Starts With Food* (Victory Belt Publishing). Check out this fantastic elevator pitch and see whether it resonates with you:

> "We eat real food — fresh, natural food, like meat, vegetables, and fruit. We choose foods that are nutrient-dense, with lots of naturally occurring vitamins and minerals, over foods that have more calories but less nutrition. And food quality is important — we are careful about where our meat, seafood, and eggs come from, and we buy organic, local produce as often as possible.

> "This is not a 'diet' — we eat as much as we need to maintain strength, energy, and a healthy body weight. We aim for well-balanced nutrition, so we eat both plants and animals. We get all the carbohydrates we need from vegetables and fruits, while healthy fats like avocado, coconut, and olive oil provide us with another excellent source of energy.

> "Eating like this allows us to maintain a healthy metabolism and keeps our immune system in balance. It's good for body composition, energy levels, sleep quality, mood, attention span, and quality of life. It helps eliminate sugar cravings and reestablishes a healthy relationship with food. It also works to minimize our risk for most lifestyle-related diseases and conditions, like diabetes, cardiovascular disease, stroke, and autoimmune conditions."

✒ **I have intestinal issues, and vegetables bother me. Can I still do the Reset?** Yes! You just need to modify a bit until your intestinal strength builds up. Low-grade intestinal ailments such as bloating, discomfort, or gas are often a signal that you need to nourish and rebuild your intestinal wall. You may have to cook your vegetables thoroughly, at least until your body transitions. You want all the fiber content the veggies provide, but you also want to almost predigest them as much as possible by chopping them into small pieces and chewing them well. Adding veggies to slow cooker dishes, soups, or stews also makes the produce easier to digest. Hold off on the raw vegetables until your body's intestinal walls start to heal and fresh, healthy cells start moving in. Eat very little fruit (raw or cooked) until your body has fully transitioned into its healing phase. Stay away from dried fruit altogether for a few months until your intestines have the digestive strength.

If you have a more serious condition such as ulcerative colitis, Crohn's disease, or inflammatory bowel disease (IBD), a few foods may cause these inflammatory intestinal conditions to become irritated. Apply the same suggestions for cooking and eating vegetables in the preceding paragraph. You may also want to avoid any fruit that you can't peel because the exterior of the fruit may cause too much roughage for your body to handle until the healing phase gains traction.

You should also avoid nuts, seeds, and all nut butters, especially if you have irritable bowel syndrome (IBS), diverticulosis, or similar inflammatory disorders. The size and shape of the nuts and seeds are very irritating to inflammatory pockets in the gut.

✒ **I have an autoimmune disease. Can I do the Reset?** Yes. If you have an autoimmune disease — such as MS, colitis, arthritis, Crohn's disease, diabetes, psoriasis, lupus, Graves' disease, or alopecia — many Paleo foods can naturally and dramatically reduce inflammation and any symptoms you may have.

However, some of the Paleo-approved foods may be a bit irritating to you, so listen to your body and remove the following if necessary:

- Eggs (whole and egg whites)

- Nightshade foods: tomatoes, hot and sweet peppers, eggplant, tomatillos, and spicy foods or spices — curry powder, crushed red pepper, chili powder, cayenne, and so on

- All dairy products (including clarified butter or ghee)

- Nuts and seeds

✒ **I have a chronic disease. Can I do the Reset?** Any chronic disease, such as cancer, heart disease, diabetes, obesity, or blood sugar issues, is perfectly suited for resetting for a Paleo diet.

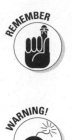

The only dietary modification here is in the case of people with diabetes. Please go slowly. Give your body time to adjust to the changes and reca-librate. Start transitioning by trading off one unhealthy meal (such breakfast) for a healthier Paleo meal and work your way up to all three meals and snacks. Be sure to create balanced meals, and make sure you are getting enough food.

I highly recommend that you work closely with a health care provider who knows you and your situation. Talk to her before you even start so you can work together as a team to adjust your insulin dose or oral medication to accommodate your new eating habits. You'll find you're going to amaze the entire office!

Chapter 5

Stocking Your Cave Kitchen

In This Chapter

▶ Giving your kitchen a Paleo overhaul

▶ Restocking your kitchen to become Paleo smart

▶ Identifying essential Paleo-approved cooking methods

The most important thing you can do to make living Paleo stick is to get your fanny in the kitchen. Cooking Paleo meals probably isn't as hard or as time consuming as you may think, so don't let this misconception get in the way of your success. I can completely relate to the time issue. I have kids, I work full time, and I'm an author to boot, so I know from experience that after you learn a couple of quick dishes, you can use them as the foundation of completely different meals with just a few small tweaks.

Before you get into the kitchen, though, you have to get your kitchen into Paleo shape. Whether you're an experienced cook or just finding your way around the kitchen, in this chapter you can find advice on how to equip your kitchen with the tools you need and utilize the best Paleo-friendly cooking methods to keep you and your family well nourished.

Clearing Your Kitchen of Non-Paleo Goods

Your commitment to living Paleo begins with changing your eating habits, so it's time to create an environment for success: the Paleo kitchen.

I have patients all the time asking for a detox to cleanse their bodies so they work more efficiently. Well, think of creating a Paleo-smart kitchen in the same way: You're cleansing your kitchen so it works more efficiently for you and your family. It may be a little uncomfortable at first, but when you're on the other side, you'll have an uncluttered food life and love how you feel.

Look at your calendar and pick a day to give your kitchen a Paleo cleanout. If you wait too long, you'll lose your momentum, so plan time soon. And actually mark it in your calendar because when you schedule something, it becomes real. Otherwise, it's just a thought.

When you first walk in your kitchen to make the Paleo transformation, take a long, hard look. Now visualize your kitchen filled with Paleo-approved foods that provide you and your family with deep nutrition. Foods that help you lose weight, boost immunity, and fight aging. Take a moment to experience how that feels in your body. Then put on some music you love and get yourself into a happy state.

I've watched people make the Paleo conversion many times, and keeping food "just in case" is a red flag. This book is filled with strategies for success, and keeping non-Paleo foods hanging around while you're trying to make the switch isn't a good strategy.

Cleansing the pantry

Open those pantry doors and just do it! As the late motivational speaker Zig Ziglar said, if you keep doing what you're doing, you'll keep getting what you're getting. Well, you're not going to be getting what you've been getting anymore. If you've been tired, battled certain health conditions, or struggled with your weight or you just want to look and feel your best, here's where you start.

Grab a trash bag and a box. The trash bag is obvious; the box is so that you set aside unopened foods to donate to your local food bank or shelter. Some people in your community are striving for calories, and you can help them by sending over a care package of your unopened non-Paleo foods.

Check the labels on your pantry items as you sort them to confirm whether they're keepable, but just a fair warning that you'll have to give most the heave-ho.

Say goodbye to the following:

- ✔ Foods with flour, including breads, pasta, crackers, chips, and cookies.
- ✔ Breakfast cereals, including granola and oatmeal.
- ✔ Foods with grains and whole grains, including wheat, barley, rye, oats, spelt, corn, and quinoa.
- ✔ Refined processed fats, such as margarine; vegetable shortening; and canola (rapeseed), soybean, grapeseed, sunflower, safflower, corn, vegetable, and peanut oils.

✔ Foods with hydrogenated or partially hydrogenated oils, including cookies, snack foods, and buttery spreads such as Earth Balance.

✔ Foods with artificial sweeteners, specifically Acesulfame K (Sweet One), aspartame (Equal and NutraSweet), saccharin (Sweet'N Low), sucralose (Splenda), stevia, and those containing erythritol (such as Truvia).

✔ Foods with soy, including soy, teriyaki, and hoisin sauces. Some tuna fish is packed in soy, so check labels.

✔ Commercial condiments with sugars and artificial ingredients, such as ketchup, BBQ sauce, sweet and sour sauces, and bottled salad dressings and marinades.

✔ Foods with cornstarch and other food starches.

✔ All sugars except for raw honey and pure maple syrup, dark chocolate, and cocoa powder.

Less-processed, natural sweeteners like raw honey and pure maple syrup can stay, but don't eat them during your 30-Day Paleo cleanse (which I cover in Chapter 4).

✔ Packaged processed foods, including microwavable meals or food bars (check all processed foods carefully because most have additives and gluten).

✔ Sauces, soups, and stews (most have thickened flours).

✔ Dressings (most are thickened with flour).

✔ Canned foods with sugars and additives, including canned fruits packed in syrup.

✔ Jam and jelly.

Clearing out the refrigerator and freezer

Emptying out the refrigerator and freezer can get dicey because you may feel like you're wasting the opened jars and containers. Those bottles of this and that all lined up along your refrigerator door make you inclined to think, "I'll wait to see whether this Paleo thing is really worth its salt." When these doubts strike, remember that you're cleansing your refrigerator. Keeping non-Paleo foods isn't part of the plan.

The following are the items you need to chuck:

✔ Any leftovers that aren't part of your healthy food plan.

✔ Commercial dressings and sauces.

✔ Dairy products, including butter, margarine, milk, cheese, cream, half-and-half, flavored creamers, yogurt, ice cream, and frozen yogurt.

✔ All soy frankenfoods, such as vegetarian burgers, hot dogs, and chicken nuggets. (*Frankenfoods* are processed foods that are made to look like a certain food product but are really made from wheat.) Pitch any tofu as well.

✔ Fruit juices or other sweetened beverages, including soda or teas.

✔ Lunchmeats, sausage, and bacon that contain gluten, nitrites, soy, or sweeteners.

✔ Commercial condiments with sugars and artificial ingredients.

✔ Frozen waffles, pizza, macaroni, or other frozen meals.

✔ Popsicles and frozen fruit bars with sugar and artificial ingredients.

What's left in your refrigerator should be eggs, unprocessed meats, fresh fruits, vegetables, and condiments that don't contain sugar or other artificial ingredients.

If you decide to have a sweet, you're better off going out and getting a single serving rather than keeping it in your house. That way, after you eat it, you're done, and you're not tempted by it lingering around the house.

Refilling Your Kitchen with Paleo Foods

You decided to take action and committed to a healthy life by clearing out the old and making way for the new. The foods you'll be restocking your kitchen with are full of nutrients and bursting with flavor. They're the foods your body was designed to eat. Enjoy making these foods your base and get excited about your healthy, vibrant future.

Picking Paleo-smart protein

When you read or hear that animal proteins aren't good for you, often the *quality* of that protein is what's in question, not the protein source. Factory-farmed meat is less healthy than meat from animals raised humanely and sustainably. When you can, your best option is always to get meat from organic, pasture-raised, antibiotic-free sources. In fact, if you're going to strain the food budget somewhere, protein is the place. If doing so isn't in the budget right now, though, don't stress. Buying the leanest cuts you can find, removing the skin on poultry and the excess fat on red meat before cooking, and removing and draining excess fat after cooking are great strategies for making conventional meats as healthy as possible. (Turn to Chapter 4 for more tips on improving the healthfulness of conventionally raised meat.)

The difference between grass-fed and pasture-raised really has to do with the animal. *Grass-fed* meat comes from animals that have lived on carefully managed pastures all their lives. When they are indoors during the winter, they are fed hay, but no grain whatsoever. *Pasture-raised* or *pastured* animals are omnivorous animals such as pigs and chickens that cannot exist exclusively on a diet of grass. They are kept on a fresh, clean pasture, and their diet is supplemented with some kind of grain. Bottom line: Beef and lamb are grass-fed; pigs and chickens are pastured.

Follow this advice for purchasing the best Paleo proteins your food budget allows:

- **Beef:** Grass-fed, organic beef provides you with the best balance of omega-6 fatty acid to omega-3 fatty acid ratios. In fact, when you buy grass-fed, you can eat all the fat — no need to cut or drain. Just be sure the beef you buy says both "grass-fed" and "grass-finished;" either one without the other means the cow likely wasn't exclusively fed grass.

- **Lamb:** All cuts are good; grass-fed is best.

- **Poultry:** All cuts of poultry are good. Organic, free-range, or pasture-raised is best.

- **Pork:** If you can't purchase pastured-raised pork or wild boar to avoid the toxins and omega-6 fatty acids of conventionally raised pork, choose another, cleaner protein source. If you buy organic bacon, make sure it's free of sugar, and eat it in moderation.

- **Game meats:** Game meats, such as elk, bison, duck, pheasant, and quail, are naturally low in fat and high in protein. When you can find them, they're great choices.

- **Organ meats:** Organic organ meats, such as liver, kidney, and heart, are rich in nutrition. Just keep in mind that organic and pasture-raised is your best bet. Conventionally raised organ meats can be toxic, so pass on those options if you can't find a pasture-raised source.

- **Eggs:** Organic and pasture-raised eggs provide the healthiest omega-6 to omega-3 ratios. You can tell the difference in the color of the yolk. A dark yellow yolk is the sign of a good egg.

Your healthiest choice for eggs is organic and pastured. You know the chickens were humanely and healthfully raised if the carton says "Certified Humane" or "Food Alliance Certified." Avoid "United Egg Producers Certified;" this certifier permits factory farm practices. When buying eggs, labels or cartons that read "vegetarian-fed" and "natural" have no impact on the quality of the eggs. Their titles sound like a breezy day at the farm but have no value.

✓ **Fish and seafood:** Wild-caught fish, seafood, and shellfish are healthier than farm-raised. Visit the Monterey Bay Aquarium Seafood Watch site (`www.montereybayaquarium.org/cr/seafoodwatch.aspx`) for recommendations from a trusted source.

✓ **Nitrite- and gluten-free deli meats and sausages:** Look on the label for added sugar, gluten, or other additives that can sabotage your healthy efforts. If you can't purchase quality deli meats and sausages, chose another protein; conventional choices can cause inflammation.

Grabbing Paleo-smart produce

Veggies provide you with tons of nutrients, reduce toxicity, increase fiber, and make you look better. They naturally reduce your chances of getting just about every disease — not to mention that they keep you healthy, young, and vibrant. Always try new and exciting vegetables in varying colors and fill your plate. The brighter and richer the color, the more good stuff you're giving your body. (*Tip:* Farmers' markets are great places to find veggies for experimenting.)

Fruits in moderation are an excellent antioxidant source. The healthier your body becomes, the more fruit you can tolerate without blood sugar swings.

One of the best qualities of fruit is its ability to naturally satisfy your taste for sweet while adding nutrition. However, just remember that eating some fruit is a good idea; eating gobs of it isn't. Fruit can satisfy sugar cravings, but it can also keep the sugar fits going. The fructose in fruit elevates blood sugar, so don't let the fruit displace vegetables. Vegetables first, fruit second.

I know grabbing a piece of fruit is easier than steaming some vegetables, but you'll soon find ways to grab veggies just as quickly the more you get into your new habits and into the flow of things. Purchase a container of washed greens (like the prepared greens from Earthbound Farm), pop open the lid, drizzle on some olive oil, and add some Celtic sea salt and a squeeze of lemon if you like. Boom: instant salad. For a more elaborate touch, add few sliced strawberries. It takes less than two minutes, and it's really good. If you want to go a step further and add protein into your veggies, you have a full-fledged balanced meal.

Local, organic, and seasonal produce is best. Frozen organic is a good choice as well because the produce is flash frozen, locking in all the freshness and goodness.

The Environmental Working Group (EWG; `www.ewg.org/foodnews/`) did testing on various produce items and found which have high pesticide contamination and are therefore most beneficial to buy organic:

> ✔ **Buy organic:** Apples, cherries, grapes, nectarines, peaches, pears, lettuce, raspberries, strawberries, blueberries, bell peppers, celery, carrots, kale, mushrooms, spinach

> ✔ **Organic optional:** Bananas, mangos, papaya, kiwi, pineapples, asparagus, avocado, broccoli, cauliflower, onions

The following vegetables are all Paleo-approved:

- ✔ Acorn squash
- ✔ Artichokes
- ✔ Arugula
- ✔ Asparagus
- ✔ Beets
- ✔ Bell peppers: Green, orange, red, and yellow
- ✔ Bok choy
- ✔ Broccoli
- ✔ Broccoli rabe
- ✔ Brussels sprouts
- ✔ Butternut squash
- ✔ Cauliflower
- ✔ Chile peppers
- ✔ Carrots
- ✔ Celery
- ✔ Celery root
- ✔ Cucumber
- ✔ Eggplant
- ✔ Garlic
- ✔ Green beans
- ✔ Green cabbage
- ✔ Greens: Beet, collard, mustard, and turnip
- ✔ Jalapeños
- ✔ Jicama
- ✔ Kale

- ✔ Kohlrabi
- ✔ Leeks
- ✔ Lettuce: Boston, butter, iceberg, leaf, and romaine
- ✔ Mushrooms
- ✔ Napa cabbage
- ✔ Onions
- ✔ Parsnips
- ✔ Plantains
- ✔ Radicchio
- ✔ Radishes
- ✔ Red cabbage
- ✔ Rutabaga
- ✔ Snap peas
- ✔ Snow peas
- ✔ Spaghetti squash
- ✔ Spinach
- ✔ Sprouts
- ✔ Summer squash
- ✔ Sweet potatoes and yams
- ✔ Swiss chard
- ✔ Tomatoes
- ✔ Turnips
- ✔ Watercress
- ✔ Yucca
- ✔ Zucchini

Some Paleo-approved vegetables are *nightshade* foods, and these may cause discomfort if you have joint pain, autoimmune conditions, MS, fibromyalgia, or chronic fatigue syndrome. They include bell peppers (green, orange, red, and yellow), chile peppers, jalepeños, eggplant, and tomatoes.

The following fruits have a place in your Paleo-approved kitchen:

✔ Apples	✔ Mangoes
✔ Apricots	✔ Nectarines
✔ Bananas	✔ Oranges
✔ Blackberries	✔ Papayas
✔ Blueberries	✔ Peaches
✔ Cantaloupe	✔ Pears
✔ Cherries	✔ Pineapples
✔ Dates	✔ Plums
✔ Figs	✔ Pomegranates
✔ Grapefruits	✔ Pumpkin
✔ Grapes	✔ Raspberries
✔ Guava	✔ Rhubarb
✔ Honeydew melons	✔ Strawberries
✔ Kiwi fruits	✔ Tangerines
✔ Lemons	✔ Ugli fruit
✔ Limes	✔ Watermelons
✔ Mandarin oranges	

Enjoy all fruit, but keep in mind that your healthiest options for everyday fruits are ones low in fructose, so choose berries and cherries most often. Dates in particular are very high in sugar.

Limit your consumption of dried fruit; it's easy to overeat, and it lacks the nutrition of fresh fruits while concentrating the sugars. You also have to be aware of the sulfites in some dried fruits, which are toxic. Always opt for no-sugar-added and sulfite-free dried fruit when you indulge or choose to skip it all together. Also be cautious of fruit juices and blending fruit into smoothies and sauces because they provide all the sugar of the fruit without the fiber and satiety of eating whole fruits.

Spicing things up

You can turn a mediocre dish into a hit with a splash of spice or a spice blend. You can purchase spices dried or fresh; just get your hands on spices that warm and ground you or make you come alive with energy, such as cayenne, cinnamon, curry, ginger, and peppermint.

Cayenne, chili powder, chipotle, red pepper flakes, and paprika are considered nightshades and may cause discomfort if you have joint pain, autoimmune conditions, MS, fibromyalgia, or chronic fatigue syndrome.

Allowing Paleo-smart fats

Putting healthy fats on your plate makes just about everything you do better! Fats nourish every structure and function of the body — including your very important brain. Fats also help you absorb nutrients more efficiently and keep you feeling full.

The key to choosing fats is to get the healthiest fats you possibly can. Fats are the second place on your shopping list (behind protein) I suggest spending extra money. Here are some good options:

- **Avocadoes:** These fruits provide *monounsaturated fats,* which are incredibly healthy. Add some in a salad, mash and use as a dip for veggies, or just eat with a spoon.

- **Olives:** Olives also offer monounsaturated fats and are a great snack or salad addition.

- **Butter and ghee:** Butter from grass-fed, pasture-raised cows and organic, grass-fed ghee (also called *clarified butter*) are fantastic cooking oils because they're stable at a very high heat. (You can find a recipe for making ghee in Chapter 9.)

  Any butter, even grass-fed, contains milk proteins. If you're super-sensitive to milk proteins or have a condition you're trying to heal, you may want to stick to ghee, in which the milk proteins are boiled off.

- **Coconut fats:** Incorporate coconut through coconut butter, flakes, and milk and fresh coconut.

- **Nuts and nut butters:** I recommend almonds, Brazil nuts, cashews, chestnuts, hazelnuts, macadamia nuts, pecans, pistachios, and walnuts. ***Note:*** Due to their toxin level, peanuts and peanut butter are off the menu.

> ✔ **Oils:** Try macadamia oil, avocado oil, coconut oil, olive oil, and walnut oil.
>
> ✔ **Seeds:** Pumpkin, sesame, and sunflower seeds and pine nuts are great Paleo choices.
>
> ✔ **Animal fats:** Eating animal fats can be healthy when they come from pastured-raised, grass-fed sources, such as *tallow* (beef fat), lamb fat, duck fat, and *schmaltz* (chicken fat).

These fats are damaging and cause inflammation, so kick them to the curb:

✔ Canola oil

✔ Corn oil

✔ Cottonseed oil

✔ Margarine

✔ Palm kernel oil

✔ Partially hydrogenated oil

✔ Peanut oil

✔ Safflower oil

✔ Soybean oil

✔ Sunflower oil

✔ Trans fats (hydrogenated oils)

✔ Vegetable shortening

Targeting inflammation, not fat

The latest science indicates that eating fats isn't the problem; it's the inflammation caused by eating fats refined, processed, packaged foods and unhealthy industrial oils like the ones in the nearby section "Clearing Your Kitchen of Non-Paleo Goods." Need some research? Here it is:

An analysis published in 2010 by the prestigious *American Journal of Clinical Nutrition* concluded that no relationship exists between the intake of saturated fat and incidence of heart disease or stroke. This study pooled data from 21 unique studies that included almost 350,000 people — 11,000 of whom developed cardiovascular disease — tracked for an average of 14 years. You can read more about this analysis at http://ajcn.nutrition.org/content/early/2010/01/13/ajcn.2009.27725.abstract.

Packing a Paleo-smart pantry

Time to replenish your pantry with foods that are going to get you results. See, Paleo isn't so boring! With these pantry foods in your arsenal, you can get really creative:

- Shredded coconut (great as a snack or to add sweetness to dishes).

- Unsweetened coconut milk (full-fat canned), unsweetened almond milk, and flax milk (instead of dairy).

- Canned chilies.

- Salsa.

- Fish sauce. (Red Boat brand is good.)

- Gluten-free hot sauce.

- Gluten-free mustard.

- Vinegar: Red wine and apple cider.

- Unsweetened, sulfite-free pickles.

- Unsweetened applesauce.

- Canned fish: tuna, salmon sardines, crab, or mackerel. (Vital Choice [www.vitalchoice.com/shop/pc/home.asp] is a great brand for very clean, fresh fish.)

- Gluten- and soy-free beef jerky.

- Nuts and seeds.

- Unsweetened nut butters.

- Artichoke hearts.

- Olives (read the label for additives; should have olives, water, and salt as the only ingredients).

- Unsweetened, sulfite-free dried fruits.

- Arrowroot powder (used as a thickener; substitute for conventional flour and cornstarch).

- Coconut flour (instead of conventional flour).

- Almond flour (instead of conventional flour).

- Coconut aminos (instead of soy sauce).

- Broth: Chicken, beef, and vegetable.

✔ Raw honey.

✔ Pure maple syrup.

✔ Dark chocolate with at least 85 percent cacao.

✔ Unsweetened cocoa powder.

✔ Sun-dried tomatoes.

✔ Tomato sauce. (Rao's is a good brand: www.raos.com/premium-sauces.aspx.)

✔ Tomatoes in a jar or a carton.

Tomatoes are acidic and react with the metal in the cans. The interior coating of the cans contains Bisphenol A (BPA), a nasty, estrogen-mimicking chemical that can make you sick and fat and cause infertility problems. All the companies in the industry have BPA issues in their cans, so buying jarred tomatoes is best. BPA-free tetra paks like Pomi or Trader Joe's brand are safe. My favorites are jarred organic strained tomatoes and tomato paste from Bionaturæ (www.bionaturae.com/tomatoes.html) and conventional tomatoes in tetra pak cartons by Pomi (http://pomi.us.com/home.php) or Trader Joe's brand Italian Tomato Starter Sauce.

Any and all sweeteners, artificial sweeteners, and no-calorie sweeteners (including Paleo-approved ones) can open the floodgate for more carb and sugar cravings. I've included some natural sweeteners on the pantry list, but don't let that mislead you into thinking that they're acceptable everyday indulgences. They're simply the best options for that once-in-a-while treat.

Sipping on Paleo-smart drinks

The worst thing you can do is drink liquid (specifically sugary) carbohydrates. Even if the drink is made from fruit, it lacks the fiber and the other parts from fruit that help to buffer the glycemic response of sugary juice. Paleo-approved drinks don't contain any added or artificial sugars, toxic dyes, preservatives, or fake anything — including vitamins. You can enjoy the following options while enjoying your health:

✔ Tea (green, herbal, white).

✔ Water with fruit slices (lemon, lime, orange, berries, and so on). Add mint or spearmint leaves for extra flavor.

✔ Mineral Water (Mountain Valley Spring Water is best: www.mountain valleyspring.com).

✔ Coffee (organic is best).

Cooking Smart to Retain Flavor and Nutrition

Cooking can help move you either toward or away from health, depending on how you do it. Little cooking tweaks or pointers can make all the difference in the health of your meal. This section offers some valuable pointers to get you cooking in the know.

You certainly don't have to be a gourmet chef to use healthy cooking techniques. Anyone can use these simple methods to prepare foods; they lock in high-octane flavor and provide deep nutrition.

Paleo-smart cooking methods

Even the best intentions and the healthiest ingredients can be ruined by unhealthy cooking methods. For example, breading and deep-frying those grass-fed meats doesn't exactly support your health and weight goals. To get the most out of your Paleo kitchen, you need to prepare foods in a way that doesn't demean their nutritional value. The Paleo-approved cooking methods in this section help you do just that.

No matter what method you use to cook your food, using spices and herbs is one of the best ways to add color, flavor, and aroma to your meals. Try to choose fresh herbs that are bright, have a pungent color, and aren't wilted. Always add them toward the end of cooking. If you're using dried herbs, you can add them at the earlier stages of cooking. Go ahead and experiment!

Baking

You don't have to add anything extra to food when you bake. You can just place lean meats, seafood, poultry, vegetables, or even fruits in a covered or uncovered pan or dish. The hot, dry air of your oven turns these foods into something special — without the extra calories or fat. Try baking some of the denser carbohydrates such as squash or sweet potatoes. The heat caramelizes the natural sugars, making for a delicious side dish.

Braising

When you *braise* meats, you first brown them on high heat to caramelize the outside and then slowly cook them at low heat in flavored liquid, such as water or broth, to make the meat tender and lock in all its flavors. Braise in the oven in a covered pan or on the stovetop in a heavy pot with a tight-fitting lid. Consider adding herbs, spices, and vegetables to the braising liquid and, when the meat is done, using the braising liquid to create a flavorful, nutrient-rich sauce.

Braising is a fantastic method to use for inexpensive, tougher cuts of meat because it tenderizes them the way other cooking methods can't. Cook times vary, but it's usually about 40 minutes per pound of meat.

Sautéing and stir-frying

Sautéing and stir-frying both involve quickly cooking foods in small amounts of fat over high, direct heat. *Sautéing* uses less fat than stir-frying does; you typically allow the food to brown before moving it around in the pan. *Stir-frying* uses more fat, and you move the food around in the pan more. They're both great methods for adding flavor to thinly, uniformly sliced meat and vegetables.

Roasting

Three words describe roasting: simple, healthy, and delicious. Just place a chicken or a beef roast in a pan, surround it with hearty vegetables, and put it in the oven for a few hours. The meat cooks in its natural juices, and you can simmer and strain the drippings in the bottom of the pan and turn them into a sauce.

Roasting and baking are similar methods of dry cooking, but you apply them to two different kinds of foods. You generally roast foods that have structure already, such as meat and vegetables. You typically bake foods that don't have much structure before going into the oven, such as casseroles or pies.

Slow cooking

Slow cooking just may be the most perfect way of cooking on the planet. Meats and vegetables cook on low temperatures over longer periods of time than with other cooking methods, so the meat gets tender and the flavors blend together. If you're busy and like warm, hearty meals, you'll love how the slow cooker can make just about anything while you're running around with kids, toiling at work, or just relaxing.

Chapter 18 is devoted entirely to slow cooker recipes.

Steaming

Steaming is as basic at it gets: You bring a small amount of liquid to a simmer on the stove, place the food in a basket suspended above the liquid, and cover the pot. The hot steam circulates through the pot and cooks the food. This method is a great way to really lock the nutrition into your vegetables, brightening their colors and making them inviting to eat. You can even flavor the liquid by adding seasonings to the water, which brings out even more flavor as they cook.

Poaching

To *poach* foods, slowly simmer the ingredients in a liquid (such as water, stock, or broth) until they're tender and thoroughly cooked. The food retains its shape and texture without drying out, leaving it tender and delicious. Poaching is a great way to cook fish so that it's tender and full of flavor.

Grilling

Grilling is a way to cook food over direct heat by placing the foods on a rack above a bed of charcoal or gas heated rocks.

Although grilling is certainly a warm-weather favorite and the center of many fun gatherings of family and friends, don't make it your everyday cooking method. Grilling food damages its proteins, producing carcinogens. Good evidence indicates that *heterocyclic amines* (HCAs) produced in meat cooked at high temperatures are carcinogenic. This risk increases when the meat is cooked well-done.

You can minimize your carcinogen exposure by using the following grilling tips:

- **Don't use grilling as your go-to cooking method.** Incorporate some of the other cooking methods in this chapter to your cooking repertoire.

- **Ditch the processed vegetable oils.** When using oils in marinades or directly on the grill, opt for saturated fats, which can withstand high heat without becoming rancid. Coconut oil and grass-fed butter are great options.

- **Incorporate lots of veggies.** When you eat grilled foods, pile on the vegetables. The antioxidants and phenols in them soften the impact of the mutations in the grilled meats.

- **Don't overheat.** Make sure you don't overcook or char the food, which greatly increases the carcinogens. Keep meat away from direct heat and don't let juices fall on the heat source. These juices cause flame-ups, which tend to char food.

Paleo-smart cooking essentials

After cleaning out and restocking your cabinets, fridge, and freezer, the next step is to start assessing your kitchen equipment. Having the right tools can make your time in the kitchen a pleasure. Here are some suggestions:

- Baking sheets
- Chef's knife and sharpening stone
- Colander
- Cutting board or flexible cutting mat
- Food processor or blender
- Food storage containers (glass or BPA-free plastic)
- Good meat thermometer
- Large deep baking pan
- Large sauté pan
- Large stockpot
- Large wok
- Measuring cups and spoons
- Mixing bowls
- Paring knife
- Saucepans (small and large)

Keeping healthy fats healthy: Smoke points

A *smoke point* refers to the temperature at which an oil is too hot to remain stable and starts breaking down and creating free radicals. When the oil starts to literally give off smoke, you've reached that point. You need to rinse the pan and add fresh oil. The more saturated the fat, the more stable it is and the higher temperature it can endure before becoming unhealthy.

Oils good for high-heat cooking include

- Butter and ghee
- Coconut oil
- Duck fat
- Lard (pork fat)
- Schmaltz (chicken fat)
- Tallow (beef fat)

Traveling Paleo

Traveling can be stressful, and that stress is compounded when you're worried about what you're going to eat after you arrive. However, there are ways you can make your trip Paleo, or at least Paleo-ish. Packing these foods for your trip can make a big difference:

✔ Avocadoes

✔ Sugar- and additive-free beef jerky

✔ Bottled water

✔ Coconut flakes

✔ Cooked chicken slices

✔ Cut-up veggies

✔ Fresh-cut fruit

✔ Hard-boiled eggs

✔ Nuts

✔ Paleo-approved deli meats

✔ Sea salt (Redmond Real Salt has a 4.75-ounce travel shaker)

✔ SeaSnax nori sheets

✔ Single serving packets of nut butter

✔ Steve's PaleoGoods PaleoKits (www.stevespaleogoods.com/default.asp)

A little preparation can go a long way and saves you from a lot of frustration when you get to your destination. If you find yourself completely stuck, just do your best to avoid gluten and added sugars.

Oils best to just drizzle over food or cook at very low temperatures include

✔ Avocado oil

✔ Flaxseed oil (occasional use only)

✔ Macadamia nut oil

✔ Olive oil

✔ Walnut oil

Chapter 6

Hunting for Paleo Foods

· ·

In This Chapter

▶ Exploring new and traditional places for modern hunting and gathering

▶ Getting a handle on why food quality matters

· ·

Falling in love with Paleo is easy. The food is top-notch; the recipes are fun and easy to make; and you'll lose weight, boost immunity, fight aging, improve performance, and heal conditions. What's not to love?

Like anything new, going Paleo involves a learning curve. The good news is that's it's a small one. Making the switch to Paleo starts with buying the right foods. In addition to discovering some of the Paleo yes and no foods, you also want to figure out how to sleuth your way through the grocery stores and other places you can hunt and gather.

This chapter slices through your learning curve by giving you the scoop on all the shopping outlets, such as traditional grocery stores, natural grocery stores, and big-box stores, and explaining how to get the best nutrition from your local farm or online.

Shopping Primally: Where to Go

Primal shopping is simply about putting real foods — the foods you're designed to eat — first. You become connected to your food in a whole different way when you begin to understand where your food comes from and focus more on quality. One key to Paleo success is to keep your pantry and refrigerator stocked with Paleo-approved foods help you stay on track. Chapter 5 has details on stocking a Paleo kitchen; you can find a comprehensive shopping list and tips on how to navigate the grocery store at www.dummies.com/how-to/content/how-to-create-a-paleoapproved-grocery-list.html.

You may be surprised by what you can find at traditional grocery stores these days. Let yourself adapt to your new grocery needs by also exploring natural food stores and buying from farm markets, farm stands, vegetable and meat shares, and online sources.

Traditional grocers

Finding Paleo-approved foods in traditional stores used to be a royal pain. But because most areas have seen increased demand for organic produce, many stores are carrying at least some organic options for fruits, vegetables, and Paleo-approved pantry items. I was shocked when visiting a small suburban grocery store to find that it actually carried grass-fed meat! If your local store doesn't stock what you're looking for, make a request; often, stores will make an effort to carry what their customers need.

To shop like a Paleo aficionado in traditional stores, following the *perimeter rule* (sticking to the outside rim of the grocery) is your best bet. The fresh produce, meat, and seafood are where you should concentrate your time in the grocery store, and those items are stocked around the perimeter

Here are some more tips for getting the most Paleo bang out of your conventional grocery's aisles:

- **Produce department:** This area is where you'll find a great deal of your shopping list. Go for rainbow colors when choosing vegetables, and give a new vegetable a shot every once in a while. Simply choose an in-season vegetable that you may have never tried before.

  Corn and white potatoes aren't Paleo-approved produce. Corn is actually a grain, and white potatoes contain *antinutrients* (substances that inhibit your ability to absorb nutrients), in addition to giving you an unfavorable blood sugar spike.

  Though all fruits are okay, your best choices are the ones lowest in fructose, including berries, cherries, avocadoes, lemons, and limes.

- **Meat and seafood:** Stick to the Paleo-approved protein lists in Chapter 5 and avoid the crop of meat invaders that are often processed.

- **Middle aisles:** The Paleo-approved pantry list in Chapter 5 is your treasure map here. Get what you need and get out of those middle aisles to resist temptation.

Big-box stores

Big-box stores used to be synonymous with cheap everything — including food. Times have really shifted here. Many of the big-box membership stores are really getting into healthier food selections. In fact, these stores are great places to stock up.

Of course, the location and the season matters, but here are some of the high-quality, Paleo-approved foods I have scored at big-box outlets:

- Almond butter
- Avocadoes
- Baby cucumbers
- Beef burgers
- Butternut squash cubes
- Canned salmon
- Chicken stock
- Coconut water
- Eggs
- Frozen berries
- Frozen meats
- Frozen salmon or salmon patties
- Frozen vegetable medleys
- Grass-fed butter
- Green tea
- Ground beef
- Healthier oils
- Lamb
- Macadamia nuts
- Marinara sauce
- Organic spinach

- ✔ Organic spring mix
- ✔ Olives
- ✔ Salsa
- ✔ Sardines
- ✔ Seasonings
- ✔ Sun-dried tomatoes

Natural/health food stores

When shopping in natural food and health food stores, stick to the perimeter and look for fresh foods such as meats, fish, eggs, and produce. Health food stores are often a wonderful place to purchase prepackaged, prewashed vegetables such as stir-fry greens, chard, or kale and even prechopped onion. These items are great time savers! In the frozen section, I purchase frozen veggies, which are great in a pinch and work well for stir-fry and slow cooker meals, as well as frozen seafood and frozen berries. The health food store is also usually a good place to purchase bulk nuts because the stock moves pretty quickly, so the nuts are typically fresh.

At natural food or health food stores, be sure you stick to Paleo proteins, carbohydrates, fats, and pantry foods. Don't get lured into grabbing the crinkly packages just because you feel "covered" because you're in a health store. The biggest trap in shopping in natural food stores is assuming that because you're in a natural foods store, what you're throwing in your basket must be healthy. Don't assume the word *organic* means "healthy." Organic foods can still be junk foods.

Community supported agriculture (CSA)

With *community supported agriculture* (CSA), you pay a seasonal fee to a farm for a share of its yield. You visit the farm once a week to get your share of vegetables; some CSAs even deliver. Many of these farms also give you the opportunity to pick some in-season produce, such as berries, or maybe even fresh wildflowers.

I have a lot of great memories of my local CSA. I took my kids there when they were little to pick up the vegetables together. The big bins of produce had signs above indicating what the weekly allotment was. We'd bring our own bags and fill them up with the vegetables.

What I like most about CSAs is that they're great way to try new vegetables. You may get a weekly share with a vegetable you've never tried before (that's how I first tried kohlrabi). Because you already paid for it, you may as well try it! You can also include the entire family in your shopping, which is a great education for the kids and a really fun family outing. It really connects them to their food and helps them grow a true appreciation for real foods. My kids have great memories of our days at the farm picking up our family farm share and picking berries.

To find a CSA near you, check out LocalHarvest (`www.localharvest.org`).

Farmers' markets

Farmers' markets are a great choice if you don't want to commit to a weekly share of vegetables with a CSA and you enjoy heading out to multiple vendors. A *farmers' market* is a community of local farmers and vendors that get together on a weekly basis to sell their products. So if you like Farmer Johnny's greens but Farmer Michael's eggs, this option is a great one-stop shop. Prices tend to be better at farmers' markets than at traditional grocery stores or natural foods markets, and sometimes you can even score eggs, meat, or poultry.

These markets are another great place to build relationships or talk about growing conditions or seasonal foods. You can get a lot of information.

Farm stands

Farm stands are a great choice if you want to get your produce from one particular farmer (as opposed to the farmers' markets in the preceding section). And unlike a CSA, which has a predetermined allotment, you get to pick exactly what you want on your own schedule (within the stand's business hours, of course). I do a lot of seminars and workshops at a local organic farm's community center. Twice a week, this farm sets up a stand where folks can come check out its fantastically fresh veggies and eggs.

If this option sounds like a good fit for you, inquire with local farms to find out whether they have farm stand hours.

Meat clubs

Meat clubs or *shares* are really useful if you like to have high-quality, fresh meat (and who wouldn't?). These shares work a lot of ways: A local farm may have a supply of grass-fed, pasture-raised meat for sale on a regular basis. Or you can you can organize a group of friends and family and go in on the purchase of a portion or even a whole animal. Some farms may even have a delivery service. Just make sure you have the freezer space to accommodate your share. I and many friends have purchased extra freezer space to accommodate meat shares because it's so worthwhile. One of the biggest bonuses of meat shares is all the money you save.

Visit Eat Wild at www.eatwild.com for a directory of farms organized by state.

Online

The Internet makes shopping for food a no-brainer; you can get so many items online that it pretty much squashes all the roadblocks to getting high-quality foods. Plus, you get delivery right to your door, which makes it incredibly easy.

I purchase some of my pantry items online. Items you may have trouble finding elsewhere, such as coconut aminos and coconut butter, are easily accessible online. Proteins and produce are easy to find online as well.

Here are some good sites to source Paleo foods and spices:

- www.eatwellguide.com
- www.eatwild.com
- www.gourmetgrassfedmeat.com
- www.grasslandbeef.com/StoreFront.bok
- www.heritagefoodsusa.com
- www.primalpacks.com
- www.pureindianfoods.com
- www.spicehound.com
- www.stevespaleogoods.com

You can also find Paleo-meal delivery businesses online. I actually started one myself called Living Paleo Foods (www.livingpaleofoods.com).

Food marketing

Food marketing can get downright evil. The amount of money corporations pour into learning exactly what type of ads consumers respond to is daunting.

Do you know what the food industry calls the *potato chip marketing equation?* This concept works off the idea that more than 90 percent of sales are made to less than 10 percent of customers. The companies figure getting existing customers to repeat buy a bag of potato chips is easier than getting a new customer to take the leap, so they study the 10 percent up and down, inside and out.

According to a 2010 Nielsen Consumer report, the average American watched more than 4 hours of TV per day, or 28 hours per week, in that year. That's two months of uninterrupted TV watching for the year! The average number of commercials the average person sees by age 65 is 2 million, and most of these commercials are ads put out by pharmaceutical companies and the food industry. Even if you don't watch TV, know that corporations pay great attention to food the packaging that you find in the stores to make sure you pick up that product.

To combat marketing, consider your food values. Getting really clear on what your foundational foods (your yes foods) are helps keep you out of the potato chip aisle. Sticking as close as you can to Paleo-approved foods makes all the ridiculous food marketing a nonissue in your life.

Focusing on Food Quality

The quality of your food can make all the difference in making Paleo work for you. You can turn an ordinary food into a superfood when you chose foods with the highest quality. What quality really means to you is you get more nutrition, which helps you build the healthiest cells possible. The following sections help you look for quality in every food category.

The best way to get quality foods is to start building relationships with people in the know. If you go to your local fishmonger, start asking what the catch of the day is. Ask what days of the week the store gets its fresh fish deliveries. The same holds true of your local butcher. These folks will usually go out of their way to help you navigate through your choices and help you get the healthiest, leanest cuts possible.

Eggs

Because eggs are such a common protein, nailing down their quality is important. Here's some help cracking egg carton labels, from most desirable to least desirable:

- **Pasture-raised:** Chickens can roam freely, and their diets consist of nutritious grasses and other plants and bugs.

- **Animal Welfare Approved:** This regulated label is a very high welfare standard reserved mostly for family farms. Chickens have continual access to shelter and pasture. No antibiotics are used.

- **Food Alliance Certified:** Chickens are uncaged and have access to the outdoors. This designation is regulated.

- **Certified organic:** Chickens are given organic feed and no antibiotics unless they're ill and require them. They must be uncaged and have some access to the outdoors. Compliance is audited.

- **Certified Humane:** Chickens are uncaged inside barns or warehouses but may or may not be kept indoors. They have space to roam freely and receive no antibiotics or hormones.

- **Free-range:** Chickens are supposed to have access to the outdoors at least 51 percent of the time. There are no restrictions on what the birds are fed and no way to verify how long they're actually roaming around outside.

- **No antibiotics/no hormones:** This label is more of a marketing ploy; these terms aren't regulated, so their validity is questionable. If you're buying eggs labeled certified organic, Animal Welfare Approved, or Certified Humane (designations that are regulated), you're still getting antibiotic- and hormone-free eggs.

- **Omega-3:** Chickens are fed fish oil or flaxseed to up the omega-3 fatty acid levels in their eggs. However, the amount isn't regulated.

- **Natural:** The term *natural* is sketchy because it isn't governmentally regulated, so it doesn't indicate adherence to any specific standard. Basically, it means the eggs are minimally processed.

- **Cage-free:** These chickens aren't roaming around freely in the great outdoors; rather, they're kept inside barns or warehouses. They have no access to the outdoors, and their living conditions vary greatly.

- **Vegetarian:** Chickens are fed a diet free of animal byproducts. However, chickens aren't naturally vegetarians, so this diet is actually contrary to their makeup.

- **American Humane Certified:** This certifier allows for both cage confinement and cage-free systems, so you have no way of knowing which environment your eggs came from.

- **United Egg Producers Certified:** This labeling is extremely misleading. The name sounds authoritative, but this certifier permits routine cruel and inhumane farm practices and caging. The label has no value whatsoever.

If you have an autoimmune or inflammatory condition such as lupus, MS, Parkinson's disease, Crohn's disease, or rheumatoid arthritis, eating eggs may irritate your condition.

Meat and seafood

Food quality is particularly important when you're dealing with protein. Getting the best-quality meats provides you with tons of nutrition. Try to start working higher-quality proteins into your budget whenever you can. If you can't afford the highest quality right now, don't beat yourself up; just remember how much good you're doing your body by getting rid of all the processed and non-Paleo foods.

Table 6-1 establishes some quality guidelines for meats; the "Best Practice" column is the ideal option, but I also provide acceptable choices for other budgets.

Table 6-1	Meat Quality Guidelines	
Best Practice	**Gold Standard**	**Okay**
Beef: Local, pasture-raised, 100% grass-fed and finished	Beef: Pasture-raised, grass-fed	Beef: Mainstream conventional, lean cuts with the visible fat trimmed
Pork: Local, pasture-raised	Pork: Organic, free-range	Pork: N/A
Poultry: Local, pasture-raised	Poultry: Organic, free-range	Poultry: Mainstream conventional

Commercial pork is simply not healthy. If you can't purchase pasture-raised or organic pork, I recommend choosing another protein.

If you want to ensure that your meat is completely grass-fed, thereby getting all the healthy fats and nutrition, make sure it's _grass-fed, finished._ This designation specifies that the cows are fattened with only grass during the last 90 to 160 days before they're processed. (Some grass-fed cattle are actually finished with grain — usually corn — during this period.) Those few months of finishing are crucial to establishing the levels of important nutrients such as conjugated linoleic acids (CLAs) and omega-3 fatty acids in the beef's animal tissues. The grain finishing process decreases those levels, which is why getting beef that's not only grass-fed but also grass-finished is important.

Finding common sense in food labels

The most important part of buying Paleo foods is buying the best quality you can afford and making sure your food is on the Paleo-approved list. Other than the Paleo-approved pantry foods in Chapter 5, buying Paleo means you'll probably be avoiding any factory produced foods with labels anyway.

If your food does have a label on it, though, you want to peek at it and make sure the food has only a few ingredients, all of which you can recognize and pronounce. After about five

ingredients, really start to scrutinize what's in the food. If it's a bunch of spices, that's fine. But the ingredient list shouldn't read like a scroll.

Beware particularly of flavor enhancers. If you see the terms *artificial and natural flavorings*, understand that these foods can include wheat, gluten, corn, and soy. Tread lightly when you see those terms. Also keep an eye out for sneaky names for foods. *Living Paleo For Dummies* (Wiley) by Melissa Joulwan and yours truly includes extensive lists on sneaky foods.

To get the leanest cuts of meat if you purchase conventional, stick to the following:

- ✔ Skinless chicken or turkey breast

- ✔ Eye of round roast or steak

- ✔ Sirloin tip or steak

- ✔ Top round roast and steak

- ✔ Bottom round roast and steak

- ✔ Top sirloin steak

- ✔ 90 percent lean or higher ground beef

To find the healthiest, highest-quality fish possible, look for *wild* (was raised and caught in the wild) or *wild-caught* fish (may have spent some time on a fish farm) or fish that was humanely harvested. For the ultimate guide, refer to the Monterey Bay Aquarium: www.montereybayaquarium.org/cr/cr_sea foodwatch/sfw_recommendations.aspx.

Produce

What's most important in the produce category is just that you eat your vegetables! You have a little more leeway with produce quality than you do with proteins and fats, but as always, quality can make a difference in nutrient and toxin levels. Here are some guidelines:

- ✔ **Best practice:** Seasonal, local, organic

- ✔ **Gold standard:** Local and organic

- ✔ **Good:** Either local or organic

- ✔ **Okay:** Mainstream conventional that's rinsed well from possible pesticides

Make sure you refer to the Environmental Working Group's Dirty Dozen and Clean 15 lists at www.ewg.org/foodnews/summary.php for a comprehensive guide to pesticides found in produce.

The store's produce manager is a great resource. Ask what's in season if you're not sure. Also, make a deal with yourself to try something new every so often; ask the produce manager if you need suggestions. This strategy really helps keep your eating from getting boring.

Fats and oils

This category is one of those places to prioritize in your budget because the right fats and oils can make your cells incredibly healthy, while unhealthy or rancid oils can cause the opposite effect. Unhealthy oils create inflammation; healthy oils help inflammation leave the body. Because inflammation is the catalyst for so many problems, adding some healthy fats in your diet really makes a big difference.

Check out these guidelines, and refer to Chapters 3 and 4 for full listings and explanations of Paleo-approved oils and fats:

- ✔ **Best practice:** Paleo-approved organic and *cold-pressed* (the temperature used in pressing doesn't decrease the quality of the oil extracted)

- ✔ **Gold standard:** Paleo-approved organic

- ✔ **Good:** Mainstream traditional Paleo-approved

Snacktime!

Here are some great no-prep, grab-and-go snack ideas:

✔ Any Paleo leftovers you can get your hands on.

✔ Apple slices with almond butter.

✔ Canned fish, such as salmon, tuna, or sardines. (For a super clean source of canned fish, check out www.vitalchoice.com.)

✔ Coconut butter. (I recommend Artisana brand: http://artisanafoods.com/products/coconut-butter.)

✔ Cold shrimp.

✔ Cold sliced meat, Paleo-approved deli meat, or grass-fed jerky.

✔ Handful of nuts.

✔ Hard-boiled eggs.

✔ Nori sheets. (I recommend SeaSnax: www.seasnax.com.)

✔ Preservative-free olives.

✔ Raw veggies with guacamole or salsa dip (Red pepper, cherry tomatoes, cucumber, kohlrabi, and jicama are my personal favorites.)

✔ Romaine lettuce hearts wrapped around leftover protein.

For more snack ideas, check out the recipes in Chapter 10.

You can add mustard, hot sauce, or salsa to any of these snacks. Just be sure to check the label and make sure your choice doesn't contain added sugar or gluten. A personal favorite is Annie's Organic Horseradish Mustard: www.annies.com/products/Organic-Condiments.

If you work out, you need to add two special snacks into your day. You should eat these snacks in addition to your regular meals.

✔ **Pre-workout fuel:** For your strongest workout, eat a small snack of protein and fat about 30 to 90 minutes before your workout if you feel that you need it. By avoiding carbs just before exercise, you help your body tap into stored fat as fuel during your workout. (Of course, this recommendation doesn't include marathons or long-duration workouts.)

✔ **Post-workout fuel:** Within 30 minutes of finishing your workout, refuel with Paleo-approved, nutrient-dense carbohydrates (such as a sweet potato or some butternut squash) along with lean protein (such as eggs, chicken breast, or salmon). Fat slows the absorption of food in your digestive system, and that usually works in your favor. Post-workout is the one time when you want to minimize fat so your muscles can quickly absorb the carbohydrates and protein they need to recover from your workout.

Part II
Simple Paleo Soups, Salads, and Snacks

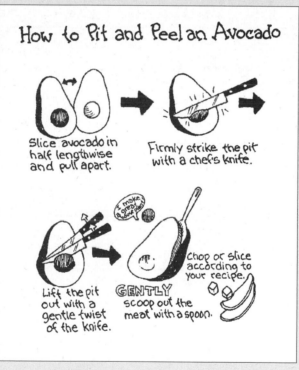

Illustration by Elizabeth Kurtzman

Find out what foods raise a red flag and should be avoided on a Paleo diet at
www.dummies.com/extras/paleocookbook.

In this part . . .

- ✔ Warm your spirit while boosting your immunity with nutrient-dense Paleo soups, a proven remedy for just about any ailment.

- ✔ Dig into the raw nutrition and fiber of Paleo salads to cleanse and create healing in your gut, which is the foundation of so much of your health.

- ✔ Whip up Paleo sauces, dressings, and salsas that make you wonder why you ever used starchy, calorie-ridden, sugary, store-bought products.

- ✔ Grab and go with energizing, nourishing Paleo snacks that aren't weighed down with sugar, carbohydrates, and additives.

Chapter 7

Savoring Comforting and Nutritious Paleo Soups

Paleo soups are a home run every time. Properly prepared soups are fantastic for their *nutritional density,* meaning they have tons of nutrition packed into their calories. Nutritionally dense foods are ideal to get a lean, strong body.

This chapter contains nine recipes for soups and broths. Broths or stocks are particularly healing because they concentrate the flavors and nutrients of their ingredients. They extract the minerals from ingredients such as vegetables in the form of electrolytes, which are easy for your body to *assimilate* (absorb) so that you build strong bones and healthy cells.

Soups are so comforting, grounding, and healing — and if you get a good bowl, you leave the table feeling as if you've had an experience. These soups are filled with flavor, easy to cook, and easy on the wallet.

Paying Attention to Ingredients

I provide recipes for great soups and broths in this chapter with the intention that you'll make them instead of buying ready-to-eat soups or broths at the grocery store. But if you find yourself in a situation where you just have to buy ready-made soup or broth, you can still ensure that you're still getting the best ingredients and none of the bad stuff.

Most canned soups contain gluten, preservatives, monosodium glutamate (MSG), and high sodium levels. Be extra careful to check labels and watch for sneaky names for wheat/gluten or MSG that often find their way into the broths:

- ✔ **Sneaky names for wheat and gluten:** If the following ingredients appear on a label, the food may contain wheat and/or gluten:

    - Artificial flavoring
    - Bleached flour
    - Caramel color
    - Dextrin
    - Flavorings
    - Hydrolyzed plant protein (HPP)
    - Hydrolyzed vegetable protein (HVP)
    - Hydrolyzed wheat protein
    - Hydrolyzed wheat starch
    - Malt
    - Maltodextrin
    - Modified food starch
    - Natural flavoring
    - Seasonings
    - Soy sauce
    - Vegetable protein
    - Vegetable starch
    - Wheat germ oil
    - Wheat grass
    - Wheat protein
    - Wheat starch

- ✔ **Sneaky names for MSG:** If the following ingredients appear on a label, the food contains MSG:

    - Any "flavors" or "flavoring"
    - Any hydrolyzed protein
    - Anything hydrolyzed
    - Anything ultra-pasteurized

- Autolyzed yeast
- Barley malt
- Calcium caseinate
- Calcium glutamate
- Carrageenan
- Citrate
- Citric acid
- Gelatin
- Glutamate
- Glutamic acid
- Magnesium glutamate
- Malt extract
- Maltodextrin
- Monoammonium glutamate
- Monopotassium glutamate
- Monosodium glutamate
- Natrium glutamate
- Pectin
- Protease
- Sodium caseinate
- Soy protein
- Soy protein concentrate
- Soy protein isolate
- Soy sauce
- Soy sauce extract
- Textured protein
- Whey protein
- Whey protein concentrate
- Whey protein isolate
- Yeast extract
- Yeast food
- Yeast nutrient

Immune-Building Vegetable Broth

Prep time: 15 min • **Cook time:** 2 hr, 15 min • **Yield:** 6 servings

Ingredients	*Directions*
6 unpeeled carrots, scrubbed and roughly chopped	*1* Put the vegetables and the garlic in a large stockpot, and add enough water to cover everything by 1 inch (about 10 cups). Cover the pot and bring to a boil.
8 stalks celery, including leafy part, roughly chopped	
2 unpeeled onions, roughly chopped	*2* Remove the lid, turn the heat to low, and simmer uncovered for about 2 hours. If the veggies start to show above the water line, add more water. Carefully skim any foam off the top as the broth simmers.
2 unpeeled large sweet potatoes, scrubbed and quartered	
1 unpeeled garnet sweet potato, scrubbed and quartered	*3* Add the cilantro, parsley, kombu, peppercorns, allspice berries, and bay leaves during the last 10 minutes of cooking. Strain the broth through cheesecloth in a large bowl.
8 cloves garlic	
1 bunch cilantro, including stems, chopped	*4* When the broth is cool, check the seasoning; add the salt and lemon juice as needed. Completely cool the broth before refrigerating or freezing.
½ cup chopped fresh flat-leaf parsley	
One 8-inch piece of kombu (seaweed)	
14 peppercorns	
4 dried allspice berries	
2 dried bay leaves	
Sea salt to taste	
Fresh lemon juice to taste	

Per serving: Calories 98 (From Fat 9); Fat 1g (Saturated 0g); Cholesterol 0mg; Sodium 115mg; Carbohydrate 23g (Dietary Fiber 5g); Protein 2.5g

Note: This broth is for healing. It's loaded with minerals and healing agents — perfect for when you have a cold or feel one coming on. You can use it as your base for all your soups to keep your immune system humming. Make a big batch and keep some in containers in your freezer; you never know when you'll need some!

Tip: Garnet sweet potatoes have darker flesh than regular sweet potatoes.

Vary It! Instead of the allspice berries and bay leaf, you can make this broth with some ginger or turmeric for a nice healing tonic. Rosemary and oregano are nice too.

This recipe has been vetted by the team at Whole9 (http://whole9life.com) and is considered acceptable for a cleansing 30-day Paleo launch.

Coconut Curry Chowder

Prep time: 15 min • **Cook time:** 25 min • **Yield:** 6 servings

Ingredients	Directions
1 onion	**1** Preheat the oven to 400 degrees.
3 small sweet potatoes	
4 tablespoons coconut oil, divided	**2** Peel and slice the onion into thin slices about 1 inch long. Chop the sweet potatoes into ½-inch cubes. Set aside.
1 teaspoon garlic powder	
1 teaspoon ground ginger	**3** Place 2 tablespoons of the coconut oil into a 9-x-9-inch baking pan and melt in the oven until the coconut oil is liquid, about 2 minutes.
1 teaspoon salt	
1 pound haddock filets	**4** Remove the pan from the oven; add the garlic powder, ginger, and salt, stirring to combine. Dip the haddock in the oil mixture so that all sides are evenly coated and bake the fish in the pan for 15 minutes.
2 tablespoons green curry paste	
2 strips bacon, cooked and chopped	
One 14.5-ounce can coconut milk	**5** While the fish is baking, add the remaining coconut oil to a medium stockpot over high heat. Add the onions and stir continuously until caramelized and translucent, about 2 minutes.
4 cups chicken broth	

6 Stir in the green curry paste and add the sweet potatoes, bacon, coconut milk, and broth. Reduce the heat to medium and simmer for 20 minutes.

7 Remove the fish from the oven and test for doneness by flaking the flesh with a fork. If it flakes easily, flake all the fish into bite-sized pieces and add them and the oil into the soup pot.

8 Stir gently for about 5 minutes and taste.

Per serving: Calories 431 (From Fat 270); Fat 30g (Saturated 24g); Cholesterol 43mg; Sodium 1,346mg; Carbohydrate 24g (Dietary Fiber 4g); Protein 20.

Tip: You can substitute another mild white fish for the haddock. I recommend the Thai Kitchen brand of green curry paste.

Recipe courtesy Audrey Olson, author of Primal Kitchen: A Family Grokumentary (www.primalkitchen.blogspot.com)

This recipe has been vetted by the team at Whole9 (http://whole9life.com) and is considered acceptable for a cleansing 30-day Paleo launch.

Turkey Spinach Soup

Prep time: 10 min • **Cook time:** 25 min • **Yield:** 4 servings

Ingredients	*Directions*
2 tablespoons coconut oil 1 medium onion, diced 2 cloves garlic, minced 1 pound ground turkey	**1** Heat the coconut oil in a large stockpot over high heat. Add the onion and garlic and sauté for 2 minutes. Add the ground turkey and sauté for an additional 7 minutes.
1 tablespoon coconut aminos	**2** Add the coconut aminos. Stir frequently for 2 minutes.
10 cups chicken broth ¼ teaspoon salt	**3** Add the chicken broth, salt, and pepper. Simmer for about 20 minutes.
¼ teaspoon pepper 4 cups fresh spinach leaves, coarsely chopped Fresh rosemary (optional)	**4** Add the spinach and rosemary (if desired) and sauté for 2 minutes. Serve.

Per serving: *Calories 347 (From Fat 126); Fat 14g (Saturated 8g); Cholesterol 81mg; Sodium 650mg; Carbohydrate 6g (Dietary Fiber 1.5g); Protein 50g.*

*Recipe courtesy Audrey Olson, author of Primal Kitchen: A Family Grokumentary (*www.primalkitchen.blogspot.com*)*

*This recipe has been vetted by the team at Whole9 (*http://whole9life.com*) and is considered acceptable for a cleansing 30-day Paleo launch.*

Curried Cream of Broccoli Soup

Prep time: 20 min • **Cook time:** 40 min • **Yield:** 6 servings

Ingredients	*Directions*
2 tablespoons coconut oil or ghee	*1* Melt the coconut oil or ghee over medium heat in a large stockpot. Add the leeks, onions, and shallots and sauté until softened, stirring frequently.
4 leeks, white and light green parts, washed and thinly sliced	
1 large onion, diced	*2* Add the broccoli, apple, and broth, topping off with water if the vegetables aren't fully submerged. Crank the heat to high, bring the soup to a boil, and then lower the heat and simmer for 20 minutes or until the vegetables are soft.
3 medium shallots, diced	
2 pounds broccoli florets	
¼ medium apple, diced	
1 quart Deep Healing Chicken Broth	*3* Stir in the curry powder and season with salt and pepper to taste.
1 tablespoon curry powder	
Kosher salt to taste	*4* Turn off the heat and let the soup cool slightly. Use an immersion blender to puree the ingredients into a smooth broth.
Pepper to taste	
1 cup coconut milk	*5* Stir the coconut milk into the soup until incorporated. Bring the soup back to a boil over high heat and ladle into serving bowls.

Per serving: *Calories 265 (From Fat 158); Fat 18g (Saturated 12g); Cholesterol 14mg; Sodium 104mg; Carbohydrate 23g (Dietary Fiber 7g); Protein 9g.*

*N*ote: You can find the recipe for Deep Healing Chicken Broth in Chapter 18.

Recipe courtesy Michelle Tam, author of Nom Nom Paleo (`http://nomnompaleo.com`*)*

This recipe has been vetted by the team at Whole9 (`http://whole9life.com`*) and is considered acceptable for a cleansing 30-day Paleo launch.*

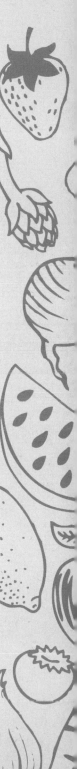

Chicken Fennel Soup

Prep time: 15 min • **Cook time:** 30 min • **Yield:** 4 servings

Ingredients	Directions
2 tablespoons ghee or grass-fed butter	*1* In a large stockpot, heat the ghee or butter over medium heat. Add the onions and chicken and sauté until the onions are translucent, about 3 minutes.
1 white onion, diced	
1 pound boneless, skinless chicken thighs or chicken breasts, chopped	*2* Add the fennel and sauté until it's softened and the chicken is partly cooked through, about 4 minutes. Add the celery, garlic, and carrots and sauté for a few minutes until fragrant.
1 fennel bulb, diced	
3 stalks celery, chopped	
3 cloves garlic, crushed	*3* Add the salt, pepper, basil, dried parsley, and stock. Bring to a boil and then simmer for 25 minutes.
2 carrots, chopped	
1 teaspoon salt	
1 teaspoon pepper	*4* Top with the fresh parsley and serve.
1 teaspoon dried basil	
1 teaspoon dried parsley	
4 cups Deep Healing Chicken Broth	
Fresh parsley for garnish	

Per serving: Calories 420 (From Fat 279); Fat 31g (Saturated 7g); Cholesterol 138mg; Sodium 630mg; Carbohydrate 6g (Dietary Fiber 2g); Protein 33g.

Note: The recipe for Deep Healing Chicken Broth is in Chapter 18.

Recipe courtesy Arsy Vartanian, author of Rubies & Radishes (www.rubiesandradishes.com)

This recipe has been vetted by the team at Whole9 (http://whole9life.com) and is considered acceptable for a cleansing 30-day Paleo launch.

Bacon Butternut Squash Soup

Prep time: 15 min • **Cook time:** 1 hr • **Yield:** 6 servings

Ingredients	Directions

Ingredients

1 large butternut squash, peeled and cut into large chunks

3 carrots, peeled and cut into large chunks

1½ tablespoons coconut oil, melted

½ pound bacon

1 small onion, chopped

1 small apple, peeled and chopped

3 cups chicken stock

1 cup coconut milk

1 teaspoon salt

1 to 2 tablespoons ground cinnamon to taste

1 tablespoon ground nutmeg

Directions

1 Preheat the oven to 350 degrees.

2 Toss the squash and carrots with the coconut oil. Arrange the mixture in a baking dish and roast uncovered for 35 minutes or until tender.

3 In a large stockpot or Dutch oven, cook the bacon over medium heat until crisp. Drain on paper towels and set aside. Sauté the onion and apple in the bacon fat until tender, about 5 minutes.

4 Add the squash, carrots, chicken stock, and coconut milk and bring to a boil, stirring often.

5 Remove the pot from the heat and use an immersion blender to blend your soup until smooth. (Alternately, you can blend the soup in a food processor or blender in several small batches and return it to the pot.)

6 Bring the blended soup to a simmer and season with the salt, cinnamon, and nutmeg. Serve in large bowls garnished with crumbled bacon or freeze and save for later.

Per serving: Calories 396 (From Fat 248); Fat 28g (Saturated 15g); Cholesterol 42mg; Sodium 1,574mg; Carbohydrate 21g (Dietary Fiber 2.5g); Protein 19g.

*Recipe courtesy George Bryant, CEO and author of Civilized Caveman Cooking Creations (*http://civilizedcavemancooking.com*)*

*This recipe has been vetted by the team at Whole9 (*http://whole9life.com*) and is considered acceptable for a cleansing 30-day Paleo launch.*

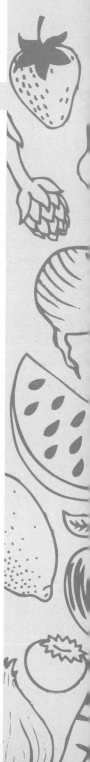

Provençal Vegetable Soup

Prep time: 20 min • **Cook time:** 30 min • **Yield:** 4 servings

Ingredients	*Directions*
1 tablespoon ghee	*1* Heat the ghee in a large stockpot. Add the leeks and sauté until soft, about 7 to 8 minutes.
2 medium leeks, white and light green parts, washed and chopped	
4 medium carrots, peeled and chopped	*2* Add the carrots, celery, and garlic and sauté until fragrant, about 5 minutes.
2 stalks celery, chopped	
4 cloves garlic, crushed	*3* Add the remaining vegetables, the vegetable stock, and the herbs. Bring to a boil and then simmer uncovered for 30 minutes or until the vegetables are tender.
2 medium zucchini, chopped	
2 medium summer squash, chopped	
6 ripe tomatoes, peeled, seeded, and chopped	*4* Salt and pepper to taste before serving.
6 cups vegetable broth	
3 sprigs fresh thyme	
¼ cup chopped fresh basil	
2 tablespoons chopped fresh parsley	
Salt and pepper to taste	

Per serving: Calories 196 (From Fat 42); Fat 4.5g (Saturated 2.5g); Cholesterol 9mg; Sodium 686mg; Carbohydrate 30g (Dietary Fiber 6g); Protein 4g.

Tip: If you can't get your hands on any fresh tomatoes, substitute jarred diced tomatoes.

Recipe courtesy Arsy Vartanian, author of Rubies & Radishes (www.rubiesandradishes.com)

This recipe has been vetted by the team at Whole9 (http://whole9life.com) and is considered acceptable for a cleansing 30-day Paleo launch.

Tomato Fennel Soup

Prep time: 20 min • **Cook time:** 30 min • **Yield:** 4 servings

Ingredients	Directions
1 tablespoon ghee	*1* Heat the ghee in a large stockpot. Add the shallots and sauté until softened, about 5 minutes.
3 shallots, chopped	
3 cloves garlic, crushed	*2* Add the garlic and fennel; cook another 3 to 5 minutes until the garlic is fragrant.
2 bulbs fennel, chopped	
8 cups chopped fresh tomatoes	*3* Add the rest of the ingredients and bring to a boil. Lower to a simmer and cook uncovered for 30 minutes.
Juice of 1 lemon	
½ teaspoon dried basil	
4 cups vegetable broth	*4* Salt and pepper to taste before serving.
Salt and pepper to taste	

Per serving: Calories 258 (From Fat 51); Fat 6g (Saturated 2g); Cholesterol 9mg; Sodium 1,283mg; Carbohydrate 44g (Dietary Fiber 8g); Protein 6g.

Tip: If fresh tomatoes aren't in season, substitute jarred diced tomatoes.

Recipe courtesy Arsy Vartanian, author of Rubies & Radishes (www.rubiesandradishes.com)

This recipe has been vetted by the team at Whole9 (http://whole9life.com) and is considered acceptable for a cleansing 30-day Paleo launch.

Summertime Watermelon Soup

Prep time: 10 min, plus chilling time • **Yield:** 6 servings

Ingredients	Directions
5 cups seeded and cubed watermelon, divided	**1** Blend 3 cups of the watermelon and 1 cup of the mango in a food processor or blender until smooth.
2 cups peeled and diced mango, divided	**2** Dice the remaining watermelon and mango into smaller pieces and stir into the puree. The soup should be chunky.
¼ cup lime juice	
3 tablespoons chopped fresh mint	**3** In a separate bowl, combine the lime juice, mint, ginger, honey, and cardamom. Add to the watermelon mixture and stir well.
1 tablespoon honey	
⅛ teaspoon ground cardamom	**4** Chill for at least 2 hours and serve.

Per serving: Calories 85 (From Fat 4.5); Fat 0.5g (Saturated 0g); Cholesterol 0mg; Sodium 2.5mg; Carbohydrate 22g (Dietary Fiber 1.5g); Protein 1.5g.

Recipe courtesy Alissa Cohen, chef and author of Living on Live Food (www.alissacohen.com)

Chapter 8

Packing Nutrition into Paleo Salads

*N*othing cleanses the body like a healthy salad. The raw nutrition, water content, and fiber blend together to act like a scrub brush for your intestines, leaving your skin glowing, your hair shiny, your eyes bright, and your body lean.

Salads' crunchy textures and flavors are also appealing; plus, salads are a great way to get in a couple of servings of vegetables. Vegetables are protective against just about every disease, and you can make salad at home in about five minutes.

If you have digestive problems like irritable bowel syndrome (IBS), inflammatory bowel disease (IBD), celiac disease, Crohn's disease, leaky gut, colitis, diverticulitis, diverticulosis, or ulcerative colitis, raw vegetables can irritate your gut. Well-cooked vegetables are a better choice for you until your gut begins to heal — and it will.

Seizing the Versatility of the Salad

Salads are one of those foods that just have to be redefined. They're far from being a boring, tasteless sidekick to a main meal. You can experiment with all different kinds of lettuce bases, like romaine, mesclun, spinach, or kale. You can spice salads up with exotic, fiery, or sweet spices and add any protein from meat to fish or eggs.

Loading up on veggies at the farmers' market

A great way to try new veggies is to experience a farmers' market. You get the freshest produce on the planet. When you shop in a traditional grocery store, the produce is several days old, but the farmers' market has super-fresh, picked-at-its-peak produce that's ripe and delicious. Another bonus: You cut out the middleman, so you save money. You'll also love building relationships with your community, which make a difference, while supporting local family farms.

Salads are also the perfect food to tote along to a picnic or potluck. You can make a bright, beautiful display with a special dressing. (For Paleo-friendly dressing options, check out Chapter 9.) I often bring the Kale with a Kick Salad in this chapter to picnics or potlucks, and it's always a hit. People are amazed the kale can taste so good, and I love the conversation it sparks about nutrition and less-familiar healthy foods.

You can find more great Paleo salad recipes online at www.dummies.com/extras/paleocookbook.

Kale with a Kick Salad

Prep time: 10 min • **Cook time:** 4 min • **Yield:** 6 servings

Ingredients	Directions
2 strips bacon	**1** In a medium skillet, fry the bacon until crispy (about 4 minutes). Transfer it to several layers of paper towels to drain, blotting slightly. Chop the bacon into small pieces.
1 cup diced avocado	
½ cup diced red onion	
1 cup diced tomato	**2** In a mixing bowl, toss all the ingredients together, squeezing and massaging the kale as you mix to wilt the kale and cream the avocado.
One 8-ounce head kale, rib removed and leaves chopped	
2½ teaspoons olive oil	**3** If possible, let the mixture sit for 30 minutes for the best flavor. Otherwise, go ahead and indulge right away!
1½ teaspoons fresh lemon juice	
½ teaspoon cayenne pepper	
1 teaspoon Celtic sea salt	

Per serving: Calories 118 (From Fat 36); Fat 7g (Saturated 1.5g); Cholesterol 3mg; Sodium 309mg; Carbohydrate 12g (Dietary Fiber 1g); Protein 4.5g.

Note: Kale provides a rich supply of disease-fighting nutrients. It also makes your skin glow and your eyes shine! Red kale is my favorite for this recipe.

Note: Celtic sea salt is a highly nutritious salt because it's unrefined and full of minerals. You can purchase it at Whole Foods or from online retailers such as Amazon or `www.celticseasalt.com`. Otherwise, any unrefined sea salt will do just fine!

This recipe has been vetted by the team at Whole9 (`http://whole9life.com`) and is considered acceptable for a cleansing 30-day Paleo launch.

Avocado and Egg Salad

Prep time: 10 min • **Cook time:** 8–10 min • **Yield:** 6 servings

Ingredients	Directions
10 eggs	**1** Place the eggs in a large pot and cover with cold water. Bring to a gentle boil and then turn off the heat and cover the pot with a lid. Let the eggs sit for 15 minutes.
2 ripe avocadoes, peeled, pitted, and diced	
1 tablespoon stone-ground mustard	**2** Drain the eggs and place in a bowl of ice water until they're cool enough to handle. Shell and dice the eggs and place them in a large bowl with the avocado. Mix together, mashing the avocado slightly.
3 tablespoons fresh lemon juice	
1 tablespoon minced fresh dill	**3** Combine the remaining ingredients with the egg mixture until mixed through. Adjust salt and pepper to taste.
2 tablespoons minced fresh parsley	
1 teaspoon paprika	
Salt and pepper to taste	**4** Top with the chopped tomatoes, if desired, and serve.
Chopped tomatoes for garnish (optional)	

Per serving: Calories 212 (From Fat 144); Fat 16g (Saturated 4g); Cholesterol 310mg; Sodium 108mg; Carbohydrate 6g (Dietary Fiber 3.5g); Protein 12g.

Tip: This avocado/egg salad is a perfect recipe for an on-the-go-breakfast, wrapped in lettuce for lunch, or as a quick snack.

Tip: I recommend the Organicville brand mustard.

Recipe courtesy Arsy Vartanian, author of Rubies & Radishes (www.rubiesandradishes.com)

This recipe has been vetted by the team at Whole9 (http://whole9life.com) and is considered acceptable for a cleansing 30-day Paleo launch.

Tuscan Spinach Salad

Prep time: 10 min • **Cook time:** 10 min • **Yield:** 4 servings

Ingredients	Directions
2 eggs	*1* Place the eggs in a saucepan and cover with cold water. Bring to a gentle boil and then turn off the heat and cover the pot with a lid. Let the eggs sit for 10 minutes.
2 cups baby spinach	
1 cup chopped fresh basil	
3 tablespoons olive oil	*2* Drain the eggs and place in a bowl of ice water until they're cool enough to handle. Remove the shells and roughly chop the eggs.
1 red onion, chopped	
1 tablespoon chopped fresh oregano	
⅓ cup lemon juice	*3* Combine the eggs and the remaining ingredients in a large bowl and serve.
2 tablespoons chopped black olives	
1 avocado, peeled, pitted, and diced	

Per serving: Calories 211 (From Fat 166); Fat 19g (Saturated 3g); Cholesterol 93mg; Sodium 87mg; Carbohydrate 8g (Dietary Fiber 3.5g); Protein 5g.

Vary It! You can substitute the hard-boiled eggs for any protein you love.

This recipe has been vetted by the team at Whole9 (http://whole9life.com) and is considered acceptable for a cleansing 30-day Paleo launch.

Curried Chicken Salad

Prep time: 25 min • **Yield:** 4 servings

Ingredients	Directions
1 pound boneless, skinless chicken breast halves, cooked and diced	*1* In a large bowl, combine everything but the avocado. Adjust salt and pepper to taste.
½ cup Paleo mayonnaise	
¼ cup dried apricots, minced	*2* Cut each avocado in half, remove the pit, and top each half with the chicken salad.
⅛ cup dried cranberries, minced	
½ a small Gala apple, diced	
2 tablespoons chives, minced	
½ stalk celery, diced	
1 tablespoon minced scallion, white part only	
2 tablespoons minced red onion	
1 teaspoon mild curry powder	
Salt and pepper to taste	
2 avocadoes	

Per serving: Calories 581 (From Fat 339); Fat 38g (Saturated 6g); Cholesterol 114mg; Sodium 263mg; Carbohydrate 22g (Dietary Fiber 7g); Protein 40g.

Tip: Check out the Paleo-friendly mayo recipes in Chapter 9.

Recipe courtesy Arsy Vartanian, author of Rubies & Radishes (www.rubiesandradishes.com)

Mango and Fennel Chicken Salad

Prep time: 20 min • **Yield:** 4 servings

Ingredients	*Directions*
2 boneless, skinless grilled chicken breasts, chopped	*1* In a large bowl, combine the chicken, fennel, scallion, and parsley.
1 small fennel bulb, finely chopped	
2 scallions, chopped	*2* Divide the spinach into 4 servings and top each with the chicken mixture, mango, and avocado.
1 tablespoon minced fresh parsley	
2 cups baby spinach	*3* Drizzle with the vinaigrette.
1 mango, chopped	
1 avocado, peeled, pitted, and diced	
Sweet and Spicy Vinaigrette	

Per serving: Calories 177 (From Fat 36); Fat 4g (Saturated 1g); Cholesterol 52mg; Sodium 100mg; Carbohydrate 15g (Dietary Fiber 4g); Protein 21g.

Note: You can find the Sweet and Spicy Vinaigrette recipe in Chapter 9.

Note: Spinach is a great source of vitamins and minerals, which keeps you in a state of nutrient sufficiency. When you're nutrient sufficient, it's like you have a protective barrier against disease and aging.

Tip: When selecting fresh spinach in the store, look for crisp, evenly colored leaves. If the leaves are still on the stalk, they shouldn't be wilted and should be free of slime and spots.

Recipe courtesy Arsy Vartanian, author of Rubies & Radishes (www.rubiesandradishes.com)

This recipe has been vetted by the team at Whole9 (http://whole9life.com) and is considered acceptable for a cleansing 30-day Paleo launch.

Simple Crab Salad

Prep time: 5 min • **Cook time:** 10 min • **Yield:** 4 servings

Ingredients	*Directions*
1 pound lump crab meat, drained and picked through	*1* Combine the crab, scallions, parsley, lemon juice, and mayonnaise in a medium bowl. Mix well.
2 scallions, thinly sliced	
2 tablespoons minced fresh Italian parsley	*2* Season with salt and pepper to taste.
1 tablespoon fresh lemon juice	
2 tablespoons Paleo mayonnaise	
Kosher salt to taste	
Pepper to taste	

Per serving: Calories 134 (From Fat 41); Fat 8g (Saturated 1g); Cholesterol 103mg; Sodium 642mg; Carbohydrate 1g (Dietary Fiber 0g); Protein 16g.

Note: You can find Paleo mayo recipes in Chapter 9.

Tip: You can assemble this quick and easy salad in no time at all; just make sure your fridge is always stocked with Paleo mayonnaise and canned crab. Serve it over salad greens or make a quick appetizer by spooning it into endive spears.

Recipe courtesy Michelle Tam, author of Nom Nom Paleo (http://nomnompaleo.com)

This recipe has been vetted by the team at Whole9 (http://whole9life.com) and is considered acceptable for a cleansing 30-day Paleo launch.

Turkish Chopped Salad

Prep time: 15 min • **Yield:** 6–8 servings

Ingredients	*Directions*
¼ **cup minced fresh parsley leaves**	*1* In a medium bowl, combine the parsley, lemon juice, garlic, cumin, paprika, oregano, and sumac (if desired). Whisk until blended and then slowly drizzle in the olive oil. Season with salt and pepper to taste.
Juice of 2 lemons	
1 clove garlic, minced	
¼ **teaspoon ground cumin**	
¼ **teaspoon paprika**	*2* Dice all the vegetables to roughly the same size — a ¼-inch dice is nice — and place in a large mixing bowl. Slice the olives and add to the bowl.
¼ **teaspoon dried oregano**	
¼ **teaspoon sumac (optional)**	
⅓ **cup extra-virgin olive oil**	*3* Pour the dressing over the salad and toss until the vegetables are coated. Taste and adjust seasonings.
Salt and pepper to taste	
2 medium cucumbers, peeled	
2 medium green peppers, seeded	
3 medium tomatoes	
½ **a medium red onion**	
1 bunch radishes, tops removed	
6 ounces brined ripe black olives, drained	

Per serving: Calories 125 (From Fat 103); Fat 12g (Saturated 1.5g); Cholesterol 0mg; Sodium 166mg; Carbohydrate 6g (Dietary Fiber 1.5g); Protein 1g.

Recipe courtesy Melissa Joulwan, author of Well Fed: Paleo Recipes for People Who Love to Eat and The Clothes Make the Girl (www.theclothesmakethegirl.com)

This recipe has been vetted by the team at Whole9 (http://whole9life.com) and is considered acceptable for a cleansing 30-day Paleo launch.

Waldorf Tuna Salad

Prep time: 5 min • **Yield:** 2 servings

Ingredients	*Directions*
1 small Gala or Fuji apple, diced	*1* Mix the apple, scallions, nuts, and parsley with a fork in a medium bowl.
2 scallions, dark green tops only, thinly sliced	
2 tablespoons coarsely chopped pecans	*2* Add the tuna, mashing with the fork to break up the tuna until no big chunks remain.
1 tablespoon minced fresh parsley	*3* Add the mustard powder and mayo to the bowl and mix with a rubber spatula until blended. Allow the tuna salad sit for 15 minutes so the flavors meld, and then taste and adjust the seasonings.
Two 5-ounce cans wild-caught tuna in water, drained	
½ teaspoon mustard powder	
3–4 tablespoons Olive Oil Mayo	
Salt and pepper to taste	

Per serving: Calories 337 (From Fat 126); Fat 14g (Saturated 1.5g); Cholesterol 50mg; Sodium 665mg; Carbohydrate 13g (Dietary Fiber 3g); Protein 38g.

Note: The recipe for Olive Oil Mayo is in Chapter 9.

Tip: Use wild-caught tuna whenever possible. I recommend Vital Choice brand: www. vitalchoice.com/shop/pc/home.asp.

Recipe courtesy Melissa Joulwan, author of Well Fed: Paleo Recipes for People Who Love to Eat and The Clothes Make the Girl (www.theclothesmakethegirl.com)

This recipe has been vetted by the team at Whole9 (http://whole9life.com) and is considered acceptable for a cleansing 30-day Paleo launch.

Chapter 9

Spicing Up Paleo Cooking with Sauces, Dressings, and Salsas

- -

In This Chapter

▶ Going beyond counting calories

▶ Adding flavor without starch, excess calories, and sugar

- -

*Y*ou don't have to have dressings and sauces, but they sure do make the world a better place! You may think living Paleo means giving up your favorite condiments — who's ever seen a picture of a caveman eating mayo? — but that's just not true.

You can still have a hamburger dripping with mayonnaise or douse your eggs with ketchup if you please; you just have to redefine your mayo and ketchup by making them Paleo-style. When you make Paleo dressings and sauces with wholesome, nutritious ingredients, you're free to indulge. The recipes in this chapter are nothing like your traditional store-bought products made from starchy, sugary, artificial ingredients. They're made from real foods.

Whether your pleasure is basic condiments, dipping sauces, pesto, or even succulent salsa, you've come to the right place. These recipes give you all the taste without any of the refined junk.

Separating Good Calories from Bad

If you shy away from luscious extras like sauces and dressings because you fear those extra calories, think about this: All calories aren't created equal. The most-fattening foods in the grocery store aren't the ones with the most calories; they're the ones that wreak havoc on your blood sugar and insulin levels — the really poor-quality carbohydrates. When you eat Paleo-approved foods made from high-quality, real ingredients, you don't get that intense, constant insulin spike.

The point to grab onto is that the number of calories you consume is less important than the quality of the calories. Cutting out Paleo-friendly sauces and dressings is less productive than watching your intake of grains, fruit juices, and all that processed food in crinkly colorful packages.

Ghee

Prep time: 5 min • **Cook time:** 15 min • **Yield:** ¾ cup

Ingredients	*Directions*
1 cup unsalted butter, preferably from grass-fed cows	*1* Place a fine mesh strainer on top of a heat-safe bowl or measuring cup and tuck a triple layer of cheese-cloth in the strainer.
	2 Melt the butter in a medium pan over low heat. When the surface of the butter resembles foam and the milk solids have turned a deep golden brown (about 8 to 10 minutes), remove the pan from the heat.
	3 Carefully strain the ghee through the cheesecloth.
	4 Discard the milk solids left in the cheesecloth and store the ghee in a sealed glass jar.

Per serving (1 tablespoon): Calories 136 (From Fat 135); Fat 15g (Saturated 10g); Cholesterol 41mg; Sodium 2mg; Carbohydrate 0g (Dietary Fiber 0g); Protein 0g.

Note: Ghee is a versatile lactose- and casein-free, high-heat cooking fat that's deliciously nutty and shelf-stable for months.

*Recipe courtesy Michelle Tam, author of Nom Nom Paleo (*http://nomnompaleo.com*)*

*This recipe has been vetted by the team at Whole9 (*http://whole9life.com*) and is considered acceptable for a cleansing 30-day Paleo launch.*

Ghee: The better butter

For people who are sensitive to dairy or who've just decided to ditch dairy, choosing ghee over grass-fed butter is a smart option. *Ghee* is butter with all the milk solids removed. This elimination takes any problems you may have with dairy sensitivities off the table. The ghee recipe in this chapter is simple to make, but if you decide you want to buy some premade ghee to keep on hand when you're in a pinch, I recommend the Pure Indian Foods brand (*www.pureindianfoods.com*) because of its high standard for quality.

Moroccan Dipping Sauce

Prep time: 5 min • **Yield:** ½ cup

Ingredients

Juice of 2 lemons

1 clove garlic, minced

½ teaspoon ground cumin

¼ teaspoon sweet, hot, or smoked paprika

Pinch of ground cayenne pepper

½ teaspoon salt

¼ teaspoon pepper

⅓ cup extra-virgin olive oil

½ cup fresh cilantro leaves, minced

½ cup fresh parsley leaves, minced

Directions

1. In a small bowl, whisk together the lemon juice, garlic, cumin, paprika, cayenne, salt, and pepper.

2. Continue whisking as you stream in the oil, then stir in the cilantro and parsley.

3. Serve at room temperature or refrigerate it if you're not going to eat it within the hour. It keeps for two or three days in the fridge without diminishing its flavor.

Per serving (1 tablespoon): Calories 84 (From Fat 81); Fat 9g (Saturated 1g); Cholesterol 0mg; Sodium 148mg; Carbohydrate 1g (Dietary Fiber 0.5g); Protein 0g.

Recipe courtesy Melissa Joulwan, author of Well Fed: Paleo Recipes for People Who Love to Eat and The Clothes Make the Girl (www.theclothesmakethegirl.com)

This recipe has been vetted by the team at Whole9 (http://whole9life.com) and is considered acceptable for a cleansing 30-day Paleo launch.

Sri Lankan Curry Sauce

Prep time: 5 min • **Cook time:** 20 min • **Yield:** 2½ cups

Ingredients	Directions
2 medium jalapeño peppers, seeds and ribs removed	**1** In a blender or small food processor, blend the jalapeños, coconut, coriander, cinnamon, cumin, ginger, salt, garlic, and ¼ cup water until you have a smooth paste. Remove to a medium bowl and stir in ½ cup of the coconut milk.
¼ cup unsweetened shredded coconut	
2 teaspoons ground coriander	
1 teaspoon ground cinnamon	**2** Heat a large nonstick skillet over medium-high heat for about 3 minutes. Melt the coconut oil in the skillet and add the carrots. Sauté, stirring with a wooden spoon, until they're tender, about 3 minutes.
1½ teaspoons ground cumin	
½ teaspoon ground ginger	
¾ teaspoon salt	**3** Add the tomatoes and their juice to the carrots. Bring to a boil and then reduce the heat to simmer, stirring occasionally and crushing the tomato chunks with the back of the spoon.
2 cloves garlic, roughly chopped	
¾ cup coconut milk, divided	**4** Cook 7 to 10 minutes until the sauce thickens and the vegetables are soft.
1 tablespoon coconut oil	
3 medium carrots, grated (about 2 cups)	**5** Stir the spice paste into the tomato mixture and add the remaining coconut milk. Stir to combine, and then remove from the heat. Use immediately or store in a covered container in the refrigerator for up to one week.
Two 14.5-ounce cans diced tomatoes	

Per serving (1 tablespoon): Calories 92 (From Fat 58); Fat 7g (Saturated 6g); Cholesterol 0mg; Sodium 424mg; Carbohydrate 8g (Dietary Fiber 2g); Protein 1.5g.

Tip: Try this sauce with steamed vegetables and your meat of choice.

Recipe courtesy Melissa Joulwan, author of Well Fed: Paleo Recipes for People Who Love to Eat and The Clothes Make the Girl (www.theclothesmakethegirl.com)

This recipe has been vetted by the team at Whole9 (http://whole9life.com) and is considered acceptable for a cleansing 30-day Paleo launch.

Tangy Carrot and Ginger Salad Dressing

Prep time: 5 min • **Cook time:** 5 min • **Yield:** ¾ cup

Ingredients	Directions
½ **cup apple cider vinegar**	**1** Combine the vinegar, carrots, ginger, scallions, and mustard in a blender on high speed until liquefied. There may still be bits of carrot in the dressing, which is fine.
2 large carrots, diced	
1-inch knob of fresh ginger, peeled and sliced	
2 scallions, white parts only	**2** Add the mayonnaise and blend on low until emulsified. Add salt and pepper to taste.
1 teaspoon kosher Dijon mustard	
⅓ **cup Olive Oil Mayo**	
Kosher salt to taste	
Pepper to taste	

Per serving (1 tablespoon): Calories 48 (From Fat 40); Fat 4.5g (Saturated 0.5g); Cholesterol 7mg; Sodium 90mg; Carbohydrate 2.5g (Dietary Fiber 0.5g); Protein 0.5g.

Tip: If you prefer your dressing a bit sweeter, add a touch of honey in Step 1. You can find the recipe for Olive Oil Mayo later in this chapter.

Recipe courtesy Michelle Tam, author of Nom Nom Paleo (http://nomnompaleo.com)

This recipe has been vetted by the team at Whole9 (http://whole9life.com) and is considered acceptable for a cleansing 30-day Paleo launch.

Smooth and Creamy Avocado Dressing

Prep time: 10 min • **Yield:** ¾ cup

Ingredients	Directions
1 avocado, peeled, pitted, and cubed	**1** Blend all ingredients in a blender or food processor. Adjust the salt, cayenne (if desired), and vinegar to taste. Serve immediately.
½ cucumber, roughly chopped	
½ cup olive oil	
¼ cup honey	
3 teaspoons apple cider vinegar	
1 teaspoon Celtic sea salt	
Pinch of cayenne pepper (optional)	

Per serving (1 tablespoon): Calories 120 (From Fat 93); Fat 11g (Saturated 1.5g); Cholesterol 0mg; Sodium 107mg; Carbohydrate 7g (Dietary Fiber 1g); Protein 0.5g.

Tip: If you want the dressing to be a little more pourable, consider adding more vinegar. You can also use this dressing as-is as a veggie dip!

Tip: For the highest-quality olive oil, look for the terms *organic* and *first-pressed*.

Recipe courtesy Alissa Cohen, chef and author of Living on Live Food (www.alissacohen.com)

Paleo Ranch Dressing

Prep time: 15 min • **Yield:** 1½ cups

Ingredients	Directions
1 egg, room temperature	**1** Crack the egg into the bowl of a blender or food processor. Run it on medium speed, enough to whip the egg into a uniform mixture.
1 cup macadamia or avocado oil, room temperature	
2 teaspoons dried dill	**2** Turn the appliance onto high speed and very slowly and steadily drizzle in the oil (this process should take a few minutes).
1 teaspoon garlic powder	
1 teaspoon onion powder	
½ teaspoon sea salt	**3** After you've achieved a nice, thick mayo base, lower the speed to medium and add the remaining ingredients. If you want to be conservative, add a little of each at a time to suit your tastes.
¼ teaspoon chili powder	
¼ teaspoon ground black or white pepper	
2 tablespoons vinegar of choice	**4** Store the dressing in an airtight glass jar in the fridge and consume within a few days.
1½ teaspoons hot sauce	
1 teaspoon honey	
1 teaspoon yellow mustard	

Per serving (1 tablespoon): Calories 178 (From Fat 171); Fat 19g (Saturated 2g); Cholesterol 16mg; Sodium 104mg; Carbohydrate 2g (Dietary Fiber 0g); Protein 1.

Vary It! Omit the vinegar for thicker dressing that makes a good dip, or omit the chili powder and hot sauce if you don't want the spicy heat. If you prefer a thinner dressing, you can adjust by adding some extra vinegar. You can also vary the flavor by substituting curry paste (for tasty heat), fish sauce (for savory), or tamari and/or coconut aminos (for even more savory).

Tip: The flavor of the dressing intensifies with time in the fridge, so keep that in mind as you add your seasonings. A batch that tastes just a little underseasoned while you're making it may be just right by the next morning.

Recipe courtesy Audrey Olson, author of Primal Kitchen: A Family Grokumentary (`www.primalkitchen.blogspot.com`*)*

Sweet and Spicy Vinaigrette

Prep time: 15 min • **Yield:** ⅔ cup

Ingredients	*Directions*
½ teaspoon lemon zest	*1* Whisk together all the ingredients and serve.
⅓ cup fresh lemon juice (2–3 lemons)	
⅓ cup olive oil	
1 clove garlic, crushed	
1 teaspoon honey	
½ teaspoon Dijon mustard	
½ teaspoon minced jalapeño (optional)	
⅛ teaspoon pepper	
Salt to taste	

Per serving (1 tablespoon): Calories 62 (From Fat 58); Fat 7g (Saturated 1g); Cholesterol 0mg; Sodium 6mg; Carbohydrate 1g (Dietary Fiber 0g); Protein 0g.

Tip: Zest the lemon before juicing it.

Recipe courtesy Arsy Vartanian, author of Rubies & Radishes (www.rubiesandradishes.com)

Cilantro Vinaigrette

Prep time: 10 min • **Yield:** 1¾ cup

Ingredients	Directions
2 cups fresh cilantro leaves and stems	*1* Mix all the ingredients in a blender or food processor. Serve immediately.
1 cup apple cider vinegar	
½ cup olive oil	
1 large clove garlic	
1½ tablespoons honey	
½ teaspoon Celtic sea salt	
½ teaspoon pepper	

Per serving (1 tablespoon): Calories 41 (From Fat 36); Fat 4g (Saturated 0.5g); Cholesterol 0mg; Sodium 25mg; Carbohydrate 1.5g (Dietary Fiber 0g); Protein 0g.

Recipe courtesy Alissa Cohen, chef and author of Living on Live Food (www.alissacohen.com)

Honey Pepper Vinaigrette

Prep time: 15 min • **Cook time:** 5 min • **Yield:** 1 cup

Ingredients	*Directions*
¼ cup honey	**1** Combine all the ingredients except the oil and salt in a blender. With the blender running on medium speed, slowly drizzle in the oil to emulsify.
⅓ cup rice wine vinegar	
1 tablespoon hot pepper sauce	
½ teaspoon pepper	**2** Season with the salt to taste.
¾ cup melted coconut oil	
Kosher salt to taste	**3** Store in a squirt bottle in the refrigerator for up to one month.

Per serving (1 tablespoon): Calories 105 (From Fat 91); Fat 10g (Saturated 9g); Cholesterol 0mg; Sodium 17mg; Carbohydrate 5g (Dietary Fiber 0g); Protein 0g.

Tip: The dressing is best when brought to room temperature before using, so if you keep it in the fridge, take it out in advance.

Recipe courtesy Nick Massie, chef and author of Paleo Nick (http://paleonick.com)

Olive Oil Mayo

Prep time: 5 min, plus standing time • **Yield:** 1¼ cup

Ingredients	Directions
1 large egg	**1** Crack the egg into the container of a blender or food processor with the lemon juice and allow the liquids 30 minutes to come to room temperature.
2 tablespoons fresh lemon juice	
1¼ cup light-tasting olive oil (not extra-virgin), divided	**2** Add ¼ cup of the olive oil to the container and blend on medium speed until the ingredients are combined.
½ teaspoon dry mustard	**3** With the blender running, add the remaining olive oil in a slow, steady stream until the substance resembles traditional mayonnaise, about 2 to 3 minutes.
½ teaspoon salt	
	4 When all the oil is incorporated, transfer the mayo to a container with a lid. Mark the container with your egg expiration date — that's when the mayo expires, too.

Per serving (1 tablespoon): Calories 124 (From Fat 123); Fat 14g (Saturated 2g); Cholesterol 9mg; Sodium 62mg; Carbohydrate 0g (Dietary Fiber 0g); Protein 0g.

Note: If you're using a blender, you'll hear the pitch change as the liquid begins to form the emulsion.

Recipe courtesy Melissa Joulwan, author of Well Fed: Paleo Recipes for People Who Love to Eat and The Clothes Make the Girl (www.theclothesmakethegirl.com)

This recipe has been vetted by the team at Whole9 (http://whole9life.com) and is considered acceptable for a cleansing 30-day Paleo launch.

Cooked Olive Oil Mayo

Prep time: 10 min • **Yield:** 2 cups

Ingredients	*Directions*
2 large egg yolks	**1** Heat the egg yolk, water, and lemon juice in a small saucepan over very low heat, stirring constantly.
2 tablespoons water	
2 tablespoons fresh lemon juice	**2** At the first sign of thickness, remove the saucepan from the heat and set it in a large pan of cold water, being careful not to get water in the eggs. Continue stirring to avoid creating citrusy scrambled eggs.
1 teaspoon dry mustard	
1 teaspoon Celtic sea salt	
1 cup olive oil	**3** Transfer the egg mixture to a blender or food processor and blend for a few seconds; let it sit uncovered for at least 5 minutes to cool.
	4 Add the dry mustard and salt and blend on low speed.
	5 With the blender running, drizzle the oil slowly into the mixture until all the ingredients are combined. Scoop into a large glass container and chill immediately. The mayonnaise should keep for one week if stored correctly.

Per serving (1 tablespoon): *Calories 64 (From Fat 63); Fat 7g (Saturated 1g); Cholesterol 13mg; Sodium 40mg; Carbohydrate 0g (Dietary Fiber 0g); Protein 0g.*

Note: This recipe is great if you're wary of using raw eggs in your mayonnaise.

*Recipe courtesy Mark Sisson, author of Primal Blueprint and Mark's Daily Apple (*www. marksdailyapple.com*)*

*This recipe has been vetted by the team at Whole9 (*http://whole9life.com*) and is considered acceptable for a cleansing 30-day Paleo launch.*

Mark's Daily Apple Ketchup

Prep time: 5 min • **Yield:** 1⅓ cup

Ingredients	Directions
6 ounces tomato paste	**1** Combine all the ingredients in a food processor and blend until the onion disappears.
⅔ cup apple cider vinegar	
⅓ cup water	**2** Spoon the mixture into airtight container and store in the refrigerator.
2 tablespoons minced onion	
2 cloves garlic	
1 teaspoon salt	
⅛ teaspoon ground allspice	
⅛ teaspoon ground cloves	
⅛ teaspoon pepper	

Per serving (1 tablespoon): Calories 7 (From Fat 0); Fat 0g (Saturated 0g); Cholesterol 0mg; Sodium 167mg; Carbohydrate 1.5g (Dietary Fiber 0.5g); Protein 0g.

Recipe courtesy Mark Sisson, author of Primal Blueprint and Mark's Daily Apple (www. marksdailyapple.com)

This recipe has been vetted by the team at Whole9 (http://whole9life.com) and is considered acceptable for a cleansing 30-day Paleo launch.

Orange Coconut Marinade

Prep time: 15 min • **Yield:** ½ cup

Ingredients	Directions
1 teaspoon orange zest	*1* Mix all the ingredients in a medium bowl. Combine with meat and marinate 2 to 6 hours for best flavor.
½ teaspoon lemon zest	
Juice of 1 orange	
2 tablespoons coconut aminos	
1 teaspoon honey	
1 teaspoon grated fresh ginger	
2 cloves garlic, crushed	
¼ cup diced white onion	
½ a jalapeño, minced	
⅛ teaspoon salt	
⅛ teaspoon pepper	

Per serving (1 tablespoon): Calories 15 (From Fat 0); Fat 0g (Saturated 0g); Cholesterol 0mg; Sodium 122mg; Carbohydrate 3.5g (Dietary Fiber 0.5g); Protein 0g.

Tip: This marinade is great on chicken.

Recipe courtesy Arsy Vartanian, author of Rubies & Radishes (www.rubiesandradishes.com)

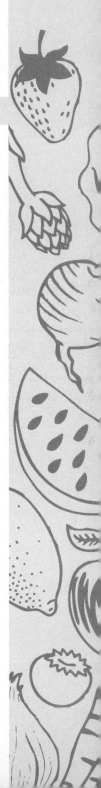

Basil and Walnut Pesto

Prep time: 5 min, plus standing time • **Yield:** 1 cup

Ingredients	Directions
2 cups fresh basil leaves, packed	*1* Combine all ingredients in a blender or food processor to desired consistency.
½ cup fresh parsley leaves, packed	
½ cup extra-virgin olive oil	*2* Allow the flavors to meld for about 30 minutes before eating. Store in an airtight container in the refrigerator.
⅓ cup walnuts	
3 cloves garlic, roughly chopped	
½ teaspoon salt	
⅛ teaspoon pepper	

*Per serving (**1 tablespoon**): Calories 80 (From Fat 76); Fat 8g (Saturated 1g); Cholesterol 0mg; Sodium 74mg; Carbohydrate 1g (Dietary Fiber 0.5g); Protein 0g.*

Recipe courtesy Melissa Joulwan, author of Well Fed: Paleo Recipes for People Who Love to Eat and The Clothes Make the Girl (www.theclothesmakethegirl.com)

This recipe has been vetted by the team at Whole9 (http://whole9life.com) and is considered acceptable for a cleansing 30-day Paleo launch.

Cucumber Avocado Salsa

Prep time: 20 min • **Yield:** 5 cups

Ingredients	Directions
2 large cucumbers, peeled, seeded, and diced	*1* Combine all ingredients except the salt and pepper in a large mixing bowl and mix well.
10 Roma tomatoes, seeded and diced	*2* Season with salt and pepper to taste.
4 limes, juiced	
2 jalapeños, minced	
½ cup chopped fresh cilantro	
2 avocadoes, peeled, pitted, and diced	
Kosher salt to taste	
Pepper to taste	

Per serving (1 tablespoon): Calories 79 (From Fat 38); Fat 4.5g (Saturated 0.5g); Cholesterol 0mg; Sodium 242mg; Carbohydrate 9g (Dietary Fiber 3.5g); Protein 2g.

Tip: For milder salsa, remove the seeds from the jalapeño before mincing it.

Recipe courtesy Nick Massie, chef and author of Paleo Nick (http://paleonick.com)

This recipe has been vetted by the team at Whole9 (http://whole9life.com) and is considered acceptable for a cleansing 30-day Paleo launch.

Tomatillo Salsa

Prep time: 25 min • **Yield:** 2⅔ cup

Ingredients

1 pound tomatillos

2 fresh poblano peppers

2 fresh Anaheim peppers

2 jalapeños

5 cloves garlic, crushed

Juice of ½ an orange

½ cup beef or chicken broth

1 teaspoon salt

½ teaspoon pepper

1 teaspoon ground cumin

1 teaspoon chipotle chili powder

½ bunch cilantro

Directions

1 Remove the husks from the tomatillos and place the tomatillos under a broiler with the poblano, Anaheim, and jalapeño peppers. Cook for 5 to 7 minutes, turning once.

2 Allow the broiled veggies to cool; remove the skins from the peppers (but not the tomatillos).

3 Blend all ingredients in a blender to the desired consistency.

4 Adjust salt and pepper to taste.

Per serving (1 tablespoon): Calories 62 (From Fat 10); Fat 1g (Saturated 0g); Cholesterol 0.5mg; Sodium 412mg; Carbohydrate 12g (Dietary Fiber 3g); Protein 2.5g.

Tip: This salsa works as a tasty topping for a Mexican-inspired salad or in the slow-cooker with chicken or beef.

Recipe courtesy Arsy Vartanian, author of Rubies & Radishes (www.rubiesandradishes.com)

This recipe has been vetted by the team at Whole9 (http://whole9life.com) and is considered acceptable for a cleansing 30-day Paleo launch.

Chapter 10

Snacking Paleo-Style

In This Chapter

▶ Keeping quick snacks handy

▶ Staying satiated with delicious Paleo snacks

*I*f three square meals a day just don't provide the fuel you need to keep going throughout your day, Paleo snacks are your answer. Paleo snacking is light-years ahead of traditional snacking. Those 100-calorie snack packs of sugary carbohydrates in attractive, crinkly packages are only masquerading as good snack choices. They aren't fuel; they're junk.

Paleo snacks fuel you with nutrient-dense foods that stabilize your blood sugar and give you lots of energy minus the bloating or fatigue other snacks can cause. Whether you're looking for the salty-sweet taste of Caramelized Coconut Chips, the protein power of quick and easy Meatball Poppers, or maybe even the simple crunch from some Roasted Rosemary Almonds, this chapter has you covered! Head to www.dummies. com/extras/paleocookbook for a recipe for Black Olive Tapenade Lettuce Rolls and other Paleo recipes that are sure to please.

There's no such thing as *junk food*. You either choose junk or choose food. You have to decide what it's going to be.

Getting the Most from One-Minute Snacks

This chapter provides you with snack recipes that are both nutritious and easy to prepare. But if you're looking for something that's a touch more grab-and-go in nature, here are some snacks that you can throw together in 60 seconds or less:

- Beef jerky and fruit
- Berries and coconut milk
- Canned fish and raw veggies
- Celery sticks and almond butter
- Leftover meat with mustard (or the Olive Oil Mayo from Chapter 9)
- Leftover protein with raw veggies or a piece of fruit
- Mashed avocado and veggies
- Olives and raw veggies
- Paleo-approved deli meat with avocado rolled up inside
- Pre-made hard-boiled eggs
- Sliced apple with nut butter
- Steve's PaleoGoods snacks, such as PaleoKits and PaleoKrunch (*www.stevespaleogoods.com*)

The best way to trip into a poor snack choice is to be starving with nothing at the ready. Be sure you have nonperishable snack items, such as nuts, sugar-free jerky, or coconut chips, available to you at all times.

Roasted Rosemary Almonds

Prep time: 5 min • **Cook time:** 8–12 min • **Yield:** 2 cups

Ingredients	Directions
1 tablespoon ghee	**1** Melt the ghee in a large skillet over medium-low heat.
2 cups whole, raw, skin-on almonds	**2** Add the almonds and stir until they're coated with ghee. Mix in the rosemary, salt, and pepper, and then shake the pan to arrange the almonds in a single layer.
2 tablespoons dried rosemary	
2 teaspoons kosher salt	**3** Toast the almonds, stirring often, until they're slightly darkened and aromatic (about 8 to 12 minutes).
¼ teaspoon pepper	
	4 Transfer to a plate and cool to room temperature. Serve right away or store in an airtight container for up to one week.

Per serving (1/4 cup): Calories 210 (From Fat 162); Fat 18g (Saturated 1.5 g); Cholesterol 0mg; Sodium 493 mg; Carbohydrate 8g (Dietary Fiber 5g); Protein 8.

Note: You can find a recipe for ghee in Chapter 9.

Tip: You can substitute fresh rosemary for a stronger, earthier flavor; adjust the quantity according to your preference.

*Recipe courtesy Michelle Tam, author of Nom Nom Paleo (*http://nomnompaleo.com*)*

*This recipe has been vetted by the team at Whole9 (*http://whole9life.com*) and is considered acceptable for a cleansing 30-day Paleo launch.*

Paleo Trail Mix

Prep time: 10 min • **Cook time:** 15 min • **Yield:** 12 servings

Ingredients	Directions
⅔ cup dried unsweetened coconut flakes (about 5 ounces)	*1* Preheat the oven to 300 degrees.
¾ cup dried unsweetened pineapple (6 ounces)	*2* Spread the coconut flakes in a single layer on a foil-rimmed baking sheet and bake for 3 to 5 minutes or until they're golden brown. Let cool.
2 cups roasted, unsalted sunflower seeds (16 ounces)	
2 cups raw, unsalted pumpkin seeds (16 ounces)	*3* Using kitchen shears, cut the pineapple into bite-sized pieces and add them to a large mixing bowl with the seeds and almonds. Add the cooled coconut flakes and mix well.
1 cup roasted, unsalted almond slivers (8 ounces)	
	4 Eat the trail mix by itself or with some coconut milk.

Per serving: Calories 378 (From Fat 279); Fat 31g (Saturated 6g); Cholesterol 0mg; Sodium 22mg; Carbohydrate 17g (Dietary Fiber 6g); Protein 14.

Tip: If you have a digital food scale, measuring out all the ingredients is a snap. Put a big bowl on the scale and weigh what you need. (Be sure to hit the "tare" button after you weigh the bowl and before you add each ingredient.)

Recipe courtesy Michelle Tam, author of Nom Nom Paleo (`http://nomnompaleo.com`)

This recipe has been vetted by the team at Whole9 (`http://whole9life.com`) and is considered acceptable for a cleansing 30-day Paleo launch.

Caramelized Coconut Chips

Prep time: 5 min • **Cook time:** 3 min • **Yield:** 1 cup

Ingredients	Directions
¼ teaspoon salt ¼ teaspoon ground cinnamon **1 cup unsweetened coconut flakes**	**1** Mix the salt and cinnamon with a fork in a small dish; set aside.
	2 Heat a skillet over medium-high heat for about 2 minutes. Add the coconut flakes and distribute evenly in a single layer. Stir frequently, continuing to spread them in a single layer, until toasted, about 3 minutes.
	3 Sprinkle the hot coconut flakes with the cinnamon mixture and toss until evenly seasoned. Transfer to a plate and allow them to cool in a single layer.

Per serving: Calories 589 (From Fat 477); Fat 53g (Saturated 48g); Cholesterol 0mg; Sodium 609mg; Carbohydrate 21g (Dietary Fiber 12g); Protein 5.

Tip: You can easily multiply this recipe to accommodate a large crowd.

Recipe courtesy Melissa Joulwan, author of Well Fed: Paleo Recipes for People Who Love to Eat and The Clothes Make the Girl (www.theclothesmakethegirl.com)

This recipe has been vetted by the team at Whole9 (http://whole9life.com) and is considered acceptable for a cleansing 30-day Paleo launch.

Sweet Potato Chips

Prep time: 5 min • **Yield:** 10 servings

Ingredients	Directions
¼ cup coconut oil	**1** Preheat the oven to 400 degrees.
2 teaspoons cayenne pepper	**2** Combine the oil and cayenne pepper in a medium bowl. Add the sweet potatoes and toss to coat them with the oil mixture.
3 sweet potatoes, peeled and thinly sliced	**3** Spread the sweet potatoes in a single layer on a parchment-lined baking sheet.
	4 Bake for approximately 20 minutes, flipping halfway through, until the sweet potatoes begin to brown. Check frequently to avoid burning smaller pieces. They will shrink in size and crisp up as they cook.
	5 Let the chips cool for about 3 minutes before serving.

Per serving: Calories 82 (From Fat 54); Fat 6g (Saturated 5g); Cholesterol 0mg; Sodium 22mg; Carbohydrate 8g (Dietary Fiber 1g); Protein 1.

*This recipe has been vetted by the team at Whole9 (*http://whole9life.com*) and is considered acceptable for a cleansing 30-day Paleo launch.*

Fried Sage Leaves

Prep time: 5 min • **Cook time:** 5 min • **Yield:** 2 servings

Ingredients	Directions
1 tablespoon ghee	**1** Heat the ghee in a medium cast-iron pan.
15 fresh whole sage leaves	**2** Place the sage leaves flat in the pan and cook until slightly crispy, only about a minute or two. Don't let them burn.

Per serving: Calories 24 (From Fat 14); Fat 1.5g (Saturated 0.5g); Cholesterol 2mg; Sodium 1mg; Carbohydrate 2g (Dietary Fiber 0g); Protein 1.

Tip: Fried sage adds a gourmet garnish to just about any dish!

Recipe courtesy Arsy Vartanian, author of Rubies & Radishes (www.rubiesandradishes.com)

This recipe has been vetted by the team at Whole9 (http://whole9life.com) and is considered acceptable for a cleansing 30-day Paleo launch.

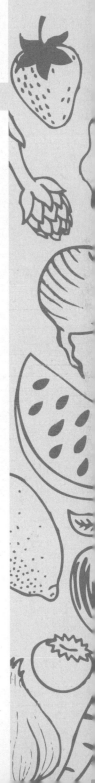

Seaweed with a Kick

Prep time: 5 min • **Yield:** 2–4 servings

Ingredients	Directions
6 nori sheets	**1** Preheat the oven to 350 degrees.
3 tablespoons melted coconut oil	**2** Spread out the nori sheets on a flat surface and rub each with ½ tablespoon of the oil. Season with the cayenne and salt.
1 teaspoon cayenne pepper	
1 teaspoon Celtic sea salt	**3** Arrange the sheets side by side on a baking sheet and bake for 3 to 4 minutes.
	4 Break the sheets into whatever size pieces you prefer and enjoy.

Per serving: Calories 95 (From Fat 90); Fat 10g (Saturated 9g); Cholesterol 0mg; Sodium 407mg; Carbohydrate 2g (Dietary Fiber 1g); Protein 1.

Tip: Nori, or edible seaweed, is definitely a smart food (I like SeaSnax brand). It's loaded with iodine, which is a trace mineral you need for healthy thyroid function. If you're not using processed iodized table salt, then you need to make sure you're getting iodine from other sources, such as this snack. Add some protein like a hard-boiled egg for a completely balanced snack!

This recipe has been vetted by the team at Whole9 (http://whole9life.com) and is considered acceptable for a cleansing 30-day Paleo launch.

Avocado Cups

Prep time: 5 min • **Yield:** 4 servings

Ingredients	Directions
2 avocadoes	**1** Halve the avocadoes and remove the pits. Use a spoon to scoop out the flesh.
2 tomatoes, diced	
½ a medium cucumber, diced	**2** In a large bowl, mash the avocado with the back of a fork and then mix in the tomatoes, cucumber, and chives. Spread this mixture into the avocado shells.
1 bunch (about 2 ounces) chives, diced	
1 tablespoon apple cider vinegar	**3** Combine the vinegar, olive oil, garlic, coconut aminos, and cayenne and pour over the avocado halves.
4 tablespoons olive oil	
1 clove garlic, minced	
½ teaspoon coconut aminos	
Dash of cayenne pepper	

Per serving: Calories 198 (From Fat 171); Fat 19g (Saturated 2.5g); Cholesterol 0mg; Sodium 21mg; Carbohydrate 8g (Dietary Fiber 4g); Protein 2.

Note: Coconut aminos are fermented coconut nectar; they're a bit like soy sauce and are a great Paleo replacement for it (because soy isn't Paleo-approved). You can find them in some traditional grocers or online at Amazon or from my favorite brand, Coconut Secret (`www.coconut secret.com/aminos2.html`).

Vary It! You can also mix some canned tuna into the avocado mixture for a more-balanced snack!

This recipe has been vetted by the team at Whole9 (`http://whole9life.com`) and is considered acceptable for a cleansing 30-day Paleo launch.

Spicy Deviled Eggs

Prep time: 15 min • **Cook time:** 15–20 min • **Yield:** 24 servings

Ingredients	Directions
12 large eggs	**1** Place the eggs in large pot and cover with cold water. Bring to a gentle boil and then turn off the heat and cover the pot with a lid. Let the eggs sit for 12 to 15 minutes.
¼ cup Olive Oil Mayo	
1 jalapeño pepper, seeded and minced	
1 teaspoon ground cumin	**2** Drain the water from the pot and transfer the eggs into a separate bowl filled with ice water until they're completely cooled. Roll each egg to crack the shell, and peel the eggs.
1 teaspoon mustard	
1 teaspoon cayenne pepper	
Paprika and salt to taste	**3** Slice each egg in half and remove the yolks, placing them in a large bowl.
1 tablespoon minced cilantro	
	4 To the egg yolks, add the mayonnaise, jalapeño, cumin, mustard, and cayenne. Add paprika and salt to taste and mix well to combine.
	5 Fill each egg white half with the mixture and garnish with the cilantro.

Per serving: Calories 45 (From Fat 27); Fat 3g (Saturated 1g); Cholesterol 94mg; Sodium 58mg; Carbohydrate 94g (Dietary Fiber 0g); Protein 3.

Note: Look for the Olive Oil Mayo recipe in Chapter 9.

Recipe courtesy Mark Sisson, author of Primal Blueprint and Mark's Daily Apple (www. marksdailyapple.com)

This recipe has been vetted by the team at Whole9 (http://whole9life.com) and is considered acceptable for a cleansing 30-day Paleo launch.

Grilled Spiced Peaches

Prep time: 10 min • **Cook time:** 15 min • **Yield:** 4 servings

Ingredients	Directions
1 tablespoon coconut oil, melted	**1** Preheat a grill on high heat.
2 teaspoons raw organic honey, melted	**2** While the grill is preheating, thoroughly mix all the ingredients except the peaches in a medium bowl.
½ teaspoon ground cinnamon	
⅛ teaspoon ground nutmeg	**3** Add the peaches to the honey sauce and toss to ensure they're evenly coated.
Pinch of chili powder	
4 white peaches, pitted and halved	**4** When the grill is warm, carefully place the peaches on the grill grates, ensuring they don't fall through. Grill for 5 minutes on each side or until they're nicely browned.
	5 Allow to cool before serving.

Per serving: Calories 100 (From Fat 36); Fat 4g (Saturated 3g); Cholesterol 0mg; Sodium 0mg; Carbohydrate 17g (Dietary Fiber 2g); Protein 1.

Tip: You can turn these peaches into a sweet treat by topping them off with any of the Paleo ice creams in Chapter 17.

Recipe courtesy George Bryant, CEO and author of Civilized Caveman Cooking Creations (http://civilizedcavemancooking.com)

Meatball Poppers

Prep time: 20 min • **Cook time:** 25–30 min • **Yield:** 12 servings

Ingredients	Directions
2 pounds ground beef	*1* Preheat the oven to 425 degrees. Line an 11-x-17-inch rimmed baking pan with parchment paper.
2 tablespoons pepper	
½ teaspoon cayenne pepper	*2* In a medium mixing bowl, combine the beef, pepper, cayenne, and chili powder. Use your hands to mix well.
½ teaspoon chili powder	
2 teaspoons coconut oil	*3* Melt the coconut oil in a large skillet over medium heat; add the onions, celery, and carrots and cook until they're translucent, about 4 minutes. Add the walnuts and sauté for an additional 2 minutes.
¼ cup minced onion	
¼ cup minced celery	
¼ cup minced carrot	
¼ cup chopped walnuts	*4* Set the onion mixture aside until it's cool enough to handle. Combine the cooled mixture with the meat and form it into 24 meatballs, roughly 1-inch in size.
	5 Place meatballs on the lined baking pan and bake 25 to 30 minutes.
	6 Serve warm with Moroccan Dipping Sauce (see the recipe in Chapter 9) if desired.

Per serving: Calories 214 (From Fat 126); Fat 14g (Saturated 5g); Cholesterol 65mg; Sodium 68mg; Carbohydrate 2g (Dietary Fiber 1g); Protein 19.

Tip: These meatballs are the best grab and go snacks! Freeze these and stock up.

This recipe has been vetted by the team at Whole9 (`http://whole9life.com`*) and is considered acceptable for a cleansing 30-day Paleo launch.*

Part III
Primal Paleo Main Dishes, Sides, and Desserts

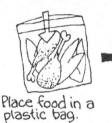
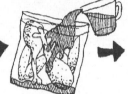
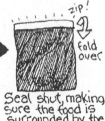
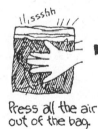

Using a Plastic Bag to Marinate Food

Place food in a plastic bag.

Pour marinade into the bag.

Press all the air out of the bag.

Seal shut, making sure the food is surrounded by the marinade, folding over if necessary.

Illustration by Elizabeth Kurtzman

web extras

Get the skinny on how to enjoy carbs relative to your activity levels at
www.dummies.com/extras/paleocookbook.

In this part . . .

- ✔ Make the most of breakfast by providing your body with high voltage nutrition and energy, and get out of the rut of having the same thing every morning.

- ✔ Prepare smarter lunches that stabilize your blood sugar and don't leave you sluggish in the middle of your busy day.

- ✔ Load up on healthy fats by preparing fresh, wild-caught fish and seafood dishes with high nutrient density.

- ✔ Pair standout proteins with other Paleo ingredients for well-rounded meat dishes.

- ✔ Take control of ingredients by making your own spice blends that are both flavorful and healing.

- ✔ Explore meat-free options with vegetarian side dishes full of vitamins, minerals, and all the best nutrients to make your body work its best.

- ✔ Reclassify desserts from guilty pleasures to homemade delights that allow you to stick to your healthy Paleo habits.

Chapter 11

Better Than Bagels: Breakfast for Living Paleo

In This Chapter

▶ Building the right kind of breakfast

▶ Fueling for the day for energy and power

How you start the day sets the tone for your entire day. Breakfast is a big piece of that puzzle. Your breakfast can either fuel you or make you feel like diving into the nearest coffeepot headfirst. If your breakfast doesn't make you feel ready to get in your zone, then you're probably not fueling right.

One of the most important Paleo principles is to dial into how food makes you feel. More than any other barometer, the mind-body connection keeps you in check. The Paleo Big Three (protein, healthy carbs, and fats) will never let you down. When you create meals by using these foods, you're golden.

Expanding Your Breakfast Options

Labels kind of box you in, and the same goes for the notion of breakfast, lunch, or dinner. So-called breakfast foods really are just food. They don't have to be granola, cereal, bagels, or anything else in a brightly colored box. A good breakfast is defined by foods that accomplish three things:

✔ Taste good while satisfying you

✔ Create a healthy blood sugar balance to prevent energy crashes

✔ Fortify you with nutrients to fuel your mind and body

Eating real foods produces these results. If you warm up a bowl of Chicken Fennel Soup for breakfast (see Chapter 7 for the recipe), you're not breaking any rules! I promise you it's not weird. As long as what you're eating satiates you, creates a favorable blood sugar balance, and fortifies your body and mind, you're good to go. You're going to get a better workout, take better care of your kids, and crush it at work or whatever you do. When you're fueling a healthy body, good stuff happens. Ditch the label "breakfast foods" and just focus on real foods for breakfast. You'll get used to it before you know it.

If you pass on most desserts because you don't want the extra sugar, you may feel duped to know that traditional breakfast cereals often have more sugar than most desserts. The Environmental Working Group's review of 84 popular cereals showed that most of them were loaded with sugar. In fact, one of the most popular kids' cereals is a staggering 56 percent sugar by weight.

If you can't fathom a breakfast without crunchy cereal and milk, mix up a batch of the Paleo Trail Mix in Chapter 10. Combine 1 cup of the trail mix with coconut milk and some berries if you like. If you want to buy pre-made trail mix, I suggest Steve's Original PaleoKrunch Cereal (which you can find at `www.stevespaleogoods.com/ProductDetails.asp?ProductCode=Cereal%2DOrig`).

Mini Cinnamon Pancakes

Prep time: 5 min • **Cook time:** 10 min • **Yield:** 12 pancakes

Ingredients	Directions
2 eggs	**1** Whisk the eggs, coconut milk, banana, vinegar, and vanilla in a medium bowl until combined.
3 tablespoons coconut milk	
3 tablespoons mashed ripe banana	**2** In a separate bowl, mix together the rest of the dry ingredients.
½ teaspoon apple cider vinegar	**3** Combine the wet and dry ingredients and mix well. The batter should be fairly thin.
½ teaspoon vanilla extract	
1½ tablespoons coconut flour	**4** Heat a tablespoon of ghee over medium heat in a small frying pan or griddle. When the fat starts sizzling, add a tablespoon of batter to the pan for each pancake. You should be able to fit three or four pancakes in the pan.
½ teaspoon ground cinnamon	
¼ teaspoon baking soda	
⅛ teaspoon kosher salt	
2 tablespoons ghee for frying	**5** Flip each pancake over when bubbles form on the surface and the edges are golden (about 1½ minutes). Cook for an additional 30 to 60 seconds on the other side.
	6 Repeat Steps 4 and 5 until you've used all the batter. (You may not need to add as much ghee each time.) Serve immediately.

Per serving: Calories 32 (From Fat 20); Fat 2.5g (Saturated 1g); Cholesterol 31mg; Sodium 63mg; Carbohydrate 2g (Dietary Fiber 0.5g); Protein 1g.

Tip: Top with fresh fruit or pureed berries for a sweet treat.

*Recipe courtesy Michelle Tam, author of Nom Nom Paleo (*http://nomnompaleo.com*)*

Almond Banana Pancakes

Prep time: 3 min • **Cook time:** 5 min • **Yield:** 2 servings

Ingredients	*Directions*
1 egg	*1* Beat the egg and mix well with the bananas.
2 ripe bananas, mashed	
1 heaping tablespoon almond butter	*2* Stir in the almond butter, adding more than a tablespoon if you want a more pancake-like texture.
1 tablespoon grass-fed butter	*3* In a large skillet, melt the butter over low heat and then pour the batter into small cakes, about 4 inches across.
	4 Brown on each side (keeping at low temperature) and serve warm.

Per serving: Calories 275 (From Fat 146); Fat 16g (Saturated 5g); Cholesterol 107mg; Sodium 50mg; Carbohydrate 29g (Dietary Fiber 4.5g); Protein 7g.

Tip: Top pancakes with grass-fed butter, fresh berries, or a touch of raw honey. Add vanilla and/or cinnamon for a delicious accent.

Note: This dish is a good option for a quick breakfast and an alternative to pancakes made with almond or coconut flour, which may be a little heavier.

*Recipe courtesy Mark Sisson, author of Primal Blueprint and Mark's Daily Apple (*www . marksdailyapple.com*)*

Morning Honey Muffins

Prep time: 10 min • **Cook time:** 15 min • **Yield:** 6 servings

Ingredients	Directions
3 eggs	**1** Preheat the oven to 400 degrees. Prepare a muffin tin by placing paper liners in 6 cups.
3 tablespoons honey	
2 tablespoons coconut oil, melted	**2** Combine the eggs, honey, coconut oil, coconut milk, salt, and vanilla.
2 tablespoons canned coconut milk	
¼ teaspoon salt	**3** Sift together the baking powder and coconut flour and then combine with the wet ingredients. Mix well and then fold in the mashed banana and chopped pecans (if desired).
¼ teaspoon vanilla extract	
¼ teaspoon baking powder	
¼ cup coconut flour	**4** Divide your batter into the lined muffin cups and bake for 15 minutes.
1 mashed ripe banana	
½ cup chopped pecans (optional)	

Per serving: Calories 160 (From Fat 86); Fat 10g (Saturated 6g); Cholesterol 92mg; Sodium 146mg; Carbohydrate 17g (Dietary Fiber 2.5g); Protein 4g.

Tip: These muffins are great with eggs or just eaten on their own. You can freeze a bunch of these for breakfast on the run.

Recipe courtesy George Bryant, CEO and author of Civilized Caveman Cooking Creations (`http://civilizedcavemancooking.com`*)*

Thai Rolled Omelet

Prep time: 5 min • **Cook time:** 10 min • **Yield:** 1 serving

Ingredients	Directions
2 eggs	**1** Crack the eggs into a medium bowl and add the fish sauce, cilantro, scallions, and a squeeze of lime juice. Whisk together until frothy.
½ teaspoon fish sauce	
1 tablespoon chopped fresh cilantro	**2** Heat the ghee in a seasoned 8-inch cast-iron skillet or a regular 8-inch skillet with sloped sides over high heat. Swirl the melted fat to cover the sides of the pan. When the ghee is shimmering, add the egg mixture.
1 tablespoon chopped scallions	
Lime wedge (¼ lime)	**3** Let the eggs sit undisturbed for 10 to 15 seconds.
1 tablespoon ghee	**4** Tip the pan back toward you at a slight angle so the omelet begins to bunch up at the far edge of the pan and then roll over itself. (You can help it roll with a spatula if needed.)
	5 When the omelet is mostly cooked through, tip it out of the pan. Serve immediately.

Per serving: Calories 211 (From Fat 135); Fat 15g (Saturated 5g); Cholesterol 372mg; Sodium 484mg; Carbohydrate 4.5g (Dietary Fiber 0.5g); Protein 14g.

Recipe courtesy Michelle Tam, author of Nom Nom Paleo (`http://nomnompaleo.com`*)*

This recipe has been vetted by the team at Whole9 (`http://whole9life.com`*) and is considered acceptable for a cleansing 30-day Paleo launch.*

Machacado and Eggs

Prep time: 5 min • **Cook time:** 10 min • **Yield:** 3 servings

Ingredients	Directions
6 eggs	**1** Crack the eggs into a medium bowl, sprinkle with the salt and pepper, and then lightly beat with a fork or whisk. Set aside.
Pinch of salt	
Pinch of pepper	
2 tablespoons coconut oil, divided	**2** Heat a skillet over medium-high heat and add 1 tablespoon of the coconut oil. When the pan is hot, add the remaining ingredients except the eggs.
¼ cup carne seca (also called machacado) or dried beef	**3** Sauté, stirring with a wooden spoon, until the onions are tender, about 7 to 10 minutes.
¼ cup diced onion	
1 clove garlic, minced	**4** Push the vegetables and beef to the side of the pan and add the remaining coconut oil. Add the eggs to the pan and push the meat into the eggs.
½ a jalapeño, ribs and seeds removed, minced	
½ a medium tomato, seeded and diced	**5** Allow the egg to begin to set, and then stir with a wooden spoon. Continue to gently scramble until the eggs are cooked to your desired doneness. Taste and adjust the seasonings.
¼ teaspoon chili powder	

Per serving: Calories 365 (From Fat 216); Fat 24g (Saturated 12g); Cholesterol 369mg; Sodium 1,180mg; Carbohydrate 6g (Dietary Fiber 1g); Protein 31g.

*Recipe courtesy Melissa Joulwan, author of Well Fed: Paleo Recipes for People Who Love to Eat and The Clothes Make the Girl (*www.theclothesmakethegirl.com*)*

*This recipe has been vetted by the team at Whole9 (*http://whole9life.com*) and is considered acceptable for a cleansing 30-day Paleo launch.*

Easy Paleo Frittata

Prep time: 5 min • **Cook time:** 20 min • **Yield:** 2 servings

Ingredients	Directions
1 tablespoon coconut oil or ghee	*1* Preheat the oven to 350 degrees.
1 cup leftover cooked meat	*2* Heat the coconut oil or ghee in an 8-inch cast-iron skillet over medium heat. Add the meat and stir-fry until heated through.
1 cup frozen broccoli or any leftover vegetables	
4 eggs	*3* If you're using frozen broccoli, place the broccoli in a microwave-safe bowl, cover it with a wet paper towel, and cook it according to the package instructions.
2 tablespoons coconut milk	
Pinch of kosher salt	
Pepper	*4* Use a pair of kitchen shears or a knife to cut the broccoli or leftover vegetables into bite-sized pieces. Add the vegetables to the meat in the pan and mix thoroughly.
	5 Crack the eggs in a medium bowl and add the coconut milk, salt, and a few grinds of pepper. Whisk well.
	6 Pour the egg mixture into the skillet and cook for 3 to 5 minutes or until the bottom of the frittata is set.
	7 Place the skillet in the oven and cook for 10 to 15 minutes or until the middle is cooked through. Set the oven temperature to broil to brown the top for a couple of minutes or until the frittata puffs up.
	8 Carefully transfer the frittata to a plate, slice, and serve.

Per serving: Calories 379 (From Fat 203); Fat 23g (Saturated 9g); Cholesterol 432mg; Sodium 263mg; Carbohydrate 7g (Dietary Fiber 3g); Protein 36g.

Tip: Throw together this easy dish with whatever leftover meat (such as sausage, seasoned ground beef, or roast chicken) and veggies you happen to have lying around. It just takes minutes to whip up a fluffy, hearty, protein-packed meal.

Recipe courtesy Michelle Tam, author of Nom Nom Paleo (http://nomnompaleo.com)

This recipe has been vetted by the team at Whole9 (http://whole9life.com) and is considered acceptable for a cleansing 30-day Paleo launch.

Eggs in Spicy Tomato Sauce

Prep time: 10 min • **Cook time:** 20–25 min • **Yield:** 3 servings

Ingredients	*Directions*
¼ **cup olive oil**	**1** Preheat the oven to 400 degrees.
3 jalapeño peppers, seeded and minced	**2** Heat the olive oil in a deep ovenproof skillet over medium heat. Add the peppers and onion and sauté until the onion is slightly browned, about 5 minutes.
1 green bell pepper, diced	
1 white or yellow onion, diced	
4 cloves garlic, minced	**3** Add the garlic, cumin, and paprika and sauté 2 minutes.
½ **teaspoon ground cumin**	
2 teaspoons paprika	**4** Add the tomatoes. Reduce the heat and simmer 15 to 20 minutes (longer if you're using fresh tomatoes), stirring occasionally, until the sauce is thickened and most of the liquid is gone. Add salt to taste.
28 ounces diced tomatoes in their juice, or 2 pounds fresh tomatoes, chopped	
Salt to taste	**5** Make 6 indentations in the veggie mixture: 5 in a circle around the skillet and one in the center. Place the skillet on the oven rack.
6 eggs	
¼ **cup chopped parsley**	
	6 Crack an egg into a small dish and carefully pour it into one of the indentations. Repeat with the remaining eggs. Close the oven and bake for about 20 minutes. Garnish with the parsley and serve warm.

Per serving: *Calories 465 (From Fat 296); Fat 33g (Saturated 7g); Cholesterol 369mg; Sodium 249mg; Carbohydrate 25g (Dietary Fiber 6g); Protein 19g.*

Note: Also known as shakshuka, this dish is loved around the world for its comforting flavor and simple preparation. (It's especially popular in Israel.) Although the sauce is often sopped up with pita bread, it's thick enough that you can skip the bread and eat it with a spoon (or spread extra sauce over leftover meat for a really fantastic meal.)

Tip: The three jalapeños make this dish pretty spicy. If you prefer less heat, use one or two instead.

Recipe courtesy Mark Sisson, author of Primal Blueprint and Mark's Daily Apple (www . marksdailyapple.com)

This recipe has been vetted by the team at Whole9 (http://whole9life.com) and is considered acceptable for a cleansing 30-day Paleo launch.

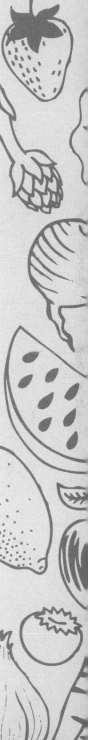

Grilled Eggs with Homemade Chorizo

Prep time: 5 min • **Cook time:** 30 min • **Yield:** 4 servings

Ingredients	Directions
2 dried ancho or guajillo chilies, stems and seeds removed ¼ cup apple cider vinegar 1 pound ground pork 1 teaspoon chili powder 1 teaspoon paprika 1 teaspoon dried oregano ½ teaspoon ground cumin ⅛ teaspoon ground cinnamon ½ teaspoon salt 2 cloves garlic, minced 2 large bell peppers 4 eggs Celtic sea salt	**1** In a dry pot heated on high, toast the chilies on each side for about 25 seconds so they start to blister. Add 2½ cups of water, bring to a boil, and then turn off the heat.
	2 Cover the pot and let the chilies soak until soft, about 30 minutes. Drain the water and blend the chilies and vinegar in a blender until a smooth paste forms.
	3 In a large bowl, mix the chili paste, pork, chili powder, paprika, oregano, cumin, cinnamon, salt, and garlic with your hands until well combined. This mixture is your chorizo sausage.
	4 Brown the chorizo in a skillet over medium heat, breaking the meat into small pieces, until it's cooked through and slightly browned on the outside, about 8 to 10 minutes.
	5 Cut the bell peppers in half through the stem. Scrape out the seeds and cut out the white membrane. Place the pepper halves on an unheated grill.
	6 Crack an egg into each pepper half and sprinkle with a handful of chorizo. Heat the grill and place the filled pepper over the hottest part of the grill to char the skin and give it a smoky flavor.
	7 Close the grill and cook for 8 to 10 minutes for a soft yolk. Check on the progress of the eggs once or twice as they cook, until they reach desired doneness.
	8 Sprinkle with Celtic sea salt and serve with extra chorizo on the side.

Per serving: Calories 337 (From Fat 132); Fat 15g (Saturated 4.5g); Cholesterol 280mg; Sodium 502mg; Carbohydrate 8g (Dietary Fiber 3g); Protein 44g.

Note: *Chorizo* is a delicious spicy Spanish pork sausage. The most important seasoning in homemade chorizo is dried chiles (ancho and guajillo are most common). Many grocery stores sell dried chiles, and you can also buy them at Hispanic markets or from online spice stores.

Tip: To help keep the bell peppers from tipping over on the grill, mold some rings out of aluminum foil to hold them upright. Place the foil rings and peppers on the cold grill, add the filling, and then turn the grill on.

*Recipe courtesy Mark Sisson, author of Primal Blueprint and Mark's Daily Apple (*www.marksdaily apple.com*)*

*This recipe has been vetted by the team at Whole9 (*http://whole9life.com*) and is considered acceptable for a cleansing 30-day Paleo launch.*

Broccoli Egg Scramble

Prep time: 5 min • **Cook time:** 5–10 min • **Yield:** 4 servings

Ingredients	Directions
2 tablespoons ghee	*1* Preheat a large skillet over low to medium heat for 1 to 2 minutes. Add the ghee, salt, and pepper.
Pinch of salt	
Pinch of pepper	
2 cups chopped broccoli	*2* Increase the heat to medium-high and add the broccoli and onion. Sauté until the broccoli is bright green but still firm, about 1 to 2 minutes.
¼ cup chopped red onion	
6 eggs	*3* While the broccoli is cooking, whisk the eggs in a medium bowl with the oregano and cayenne until well blended. Reduce the heat to medium and add the egg mixture to the pan. Let it cook without stirring right away.
½ teaspoon dried oregano	
Pinch of cayenne pepper	
2 handfuls baby spinach (about 2 ounces)	
1 ripe avocado, halved, pitted, and sliced	*4* With a small spatula, flip portions of the mixture. You'll likely only need to flip a couple of times. Don't overcook the eggs. They should remain just a little wet and in large pieces.
½ cup sliced strawberries	
	5 Divide the spinach between two plates and top with the egg mixture. Garnish each dish with the avocado and strawberries.

Per serving: *Calories 243 (From Fat 144); Fat 16g (Saturated 4g); Cholesterol 278mg; Sodium 418mg; Carbohydrate 12g (Dietary Fiber 7g); Protein 14g.*

Vary It! This recipe works with almost any combination of your favorite veggies. You may also add bacon or sausage to the pan before you sauté the vegetables for a meatier version.

Tip: Boost the flavor by adding more oregano and cayenne pepper.

*This recipe has been vetted by the team at Whole9 (*http://whole9life.com*) and is considered acceptable for a cleansing 30-day Paleo launch.*

Chapter 12

Paleo Lunches to Recharge Your System

*E*ating real food for lunch is an essential part of living Paleo. If you work from home, you can throw together simple, delicious meals at lunchtime. If you commute to an office every day, packing your lunch is usually your best bet to avoid sugary, grain-laden lunches. The key to a good Paleo lunch is doing away with the mindset that your lunch has to be just a sandwich or salad. Break the traditional lunch rules by eating nutritious foods, no matter what they are. If you're into eggs for lunch, get cracking!

If you pack your lunches, invest in toxin-free, BPA-free containers in various sizes. LunchBots are my favorite food storage containers: www.lunchbots.com.

Evolving Past Sandwiches

One of the reasons people stick to sandwiches for lunch is that they're easy to throw together, which for many is essential. The problem is that after you eat the sandwich, you feel full and lethargic — like you swallowed a bowling ball. Sandwiches aren't the only quick lunch on the block; you can easily throw together a Paleo-friendly lunch and save the bowling ball for league night.

For pain-free lunches, check out these pointers:

- ✔ **Double your dinner recipes:** If you multiply your recipes at night for dinners, you can use the leftover protein for your lunch the next day. Now just add some vegetables, fruits, and healthy fat, and your lunch is ready to go.

- ✔ **Assemble an easy Paleo soup:** Bring in a thermos of your favorite Paleo broth (see Chapters 7 and 18 for options) and a container of protein and veggies. Pour the hot broth over protein and veggies before serving.

- ✔ **Create a meal plan:** One of the ways I made my life so much easier as a working mom was to set up a two-week dinner schedule that constantly repeated. I never had any guesswork or surprises, and it made life so easy. You can apply the same approach to your lunches. Engage in a Monday through Friday schedule and rotate. For example, Mondays are stir-fry, Wednesdays are lettuce wraps, and Fridays are soups.

Paleo Chicken Wraps

Prep time: 15 min • **Cook time:** 10 min • **Yield:** 4 servings

Ingredients	*Directions*
1 head Bibb lettuce	*1* Separate the lettuce leaves and wash and dry them.
1 tablespoon coconut oil	
½ cup diced red onion	*2* In a large skillet, heat the coconut oil over medium heat; add the onions and sauté for one minute Add the chicken and cook until it's no longer pink, about 10 minutes.
1 pound ground chicken	
3 tablespoons chopped fresh cilantro	
3 tablespoons lime juice	*3* Stir in the cilantro, lime juice, fish sauce, salt, pepper, and chili powder.
1½ tablespoons fish sauce	
½ teaspoon salt	*4* Divide the lettuce leaves among four servings and spoon the chicken mixture into each lettuce leaf.
½ teaspoon pepper	
½ teaspoon chili powder	*5* Sprinkle on some coconut aminos and hot sauce (if desired).
Coconut aminos to taste (optional)	
Hot sauce to taste (optional)	

Per serving: *Calories 267 (From Fat 159); Fat 18g (Saturated 7g); Cholesterol 121mg; Sodium 908mg; Carbohydrate 5g (Dietary Fiber 1.5g); Protein 26g.*

Tip: Red Boat brand fish sauce is Paleo-approved. Coconut aminos are a fantastic replacement for soy sauce. If you like the taste of soy sauce, you may want to sprinkle some aminos on to finish off your wraps.

*This recipe has been vetted by the team at Whole9 (*http://whole9life.com*) and is considered acceptable for a cleansing 30-day Paleo launch.*

Tuna and Avocado Wraps

Prep time: 5 min • **Yield:** 1 serving

Ingredients	*Directions*
One 5-ounce can wild albacore tuna, drained	*1* Place the tuna in a small bowl and gently break apart the fish with a fork.
1 scallion, thinly sliced	
½ a medium jalapeño pepper, seeded and minced	*2* Add the scallion and jalapeño to the tuna and mix well. Add salt and pepper to taste.
Kosher salt to taste	
Pepper to taste	*3* In a separate bowl, mash the avocado with the lime juice and salt and pepper to taste. Add this guacamole to the tuna mixture and stir to combine.
½ a medium avocado, pitted and peeled	
Juice of half a lime	*4* Spoon the tuna salad onto the lettuce leaves and eat immediately.
2 butter lettuce leaves	

Per serving: Calories 299 (From Fat 105); Fat 12g (Saturated 2g); Cholesterol 43mg; Sodium 491mg; Carbohydrate 11g (Dietary Fiber 6g); Protein 39g.

*Recipe courtesy Michelle Tam, author of Nom Nom Paleo (*http://nomnompaleo.com*)*

*This recipe has been vetted by the team at Whole9 (*http://whole9life.com*) and is considered acceptable for a cleansing 30-day Paleo launch.*

Cabbage Slaw with Tangy Carrot Dressing

Prep time: 5 min, plus refrigeration time • **Yield:** 3 servings

Ingredients	*Directions*
½ **a medium head of red cabbage, thinly sliced**	*1* Combine the cabbage, carrot, cilantro, scallions, and dressing in a medium bowl and toss well.
1 medium carrot, peeled and shredded	
½ **cup fresh cilantro, roughly chopped**	*2* Let the slaw marinate in the fridge for at least 1 hour or until you're ready to serve it.
2 scallions, thinly sliced	
2 to 4 tablespoons Tangy Carrot and Ginger Salad Dressing	*3* Before serving, mix in the avocado and sprinkle with the almonds (if desired).
1 avocado, peeled, pitted, and diced	
¼ **cup toasted slivered almonds (optional)**	

Per serving: Calories 186 (From Fat 99); Fat 11g (Saturated 1.5g); Cholesterol 0mg; Sodium 75mg; Carbohydrate 21g (Dietary Fiber 9g); Protein 5g.

Note: The recipe for the Tangy Carrot and Ginger Salad Dressing appears in Chapter 9.

Tip: This slaw tastes better if you make it ahead because the cabbage softens and absorbs the flavorful dressing.

Recipe courtesy Michelle Tam, author of Nom Nom Paleo (http://nomnompaleo.com)

This recipe has been vetted by the team at Whole9 (http://whole9life.com) *and is considered acceptable for a cleansing 30-day Paleo launch.*

Scotch Eggs

Prep time: 15 min • **Cook time:** 30 min • **Yield:** 8 servings

Ingredients	Directions
2 pounds ground pork	*1* Preheat the oven to 375 degrees. Cover a rimmed baking sheet with parchment paper.
2 teaspoons salt	
1 teaspoon pepper	*2* In a large mixing bowl, combine the pork, salt, pepper, nutmeg, cinnamon, cloves, tarragon, parsley, chives, and garlic. Knead with your hands until well mixed.
½ teaspoon ground nutmeg	
Pinch of ground cinnamon	
Pinch of ground cloves	*3* Divide the pork mixture into 8 equal servings. Roll each piece into a ball and flatten it into a pancake shape. Wrap the meat around a hard-boiled egg, rolling it between your palms until the egg is evenly covered.
1 teaspoon dried tarragon leaves	
¼ cup fresh parsley leaves, minced	
1 tablespoon dried chives	*4* Place the meat-wrapped eggs on the baking sheet.
2 cloves garlic, minced	*5* If desired, place the pork rinds in the bowl of the food processor and process until they resemble bread crumbs; pour them onto a plate or in a shallow bowl. In another shallow bowl, beat the raw eggs.
8 hard-boiled eggs, peeled	
4 ounces fried pork rinds (optional)	
1 raw eggs (optional)	*6* Gently roll each wrapped egg in pork rind crumbs to get a thin dusting. Roll in the raw egg and then roll a second time in the crushed pork rinds to evenly coat. Place on the baking sheet.
	7 Bake for 25 minutes; increase the temperature to 400 degrees and bake an additional 5 to 10 minutes, until the meat balls are golden brown and crisp.

Per serving: Calories 345 (From Fat 198); Fat 22g (Saturated 8g); Cholesterol 277mg; Sodium 735mg; Carbohydrate 1.5g (Dietary Fiber 0g); Protein 36g.

Tip: Moisten your hands with a little water if the raw meat sticks to them while you're wrapping the eggs.

Note: If you use pork rinds, make sure they're all natural and contain just pork and salt — no MSG or other additives. A good brand is Carolina Gold Nuggets.

*Recipe courtesy Melissa Joulwan, author of Well Fed: Paleo Recipes for People Who Love to Eat and The Clothes Make the Girl (*www.theclothesmakethegirl.com*)*

*This recipe has been vetted by the team at Whole9 (*http://whole9life.com*) and is considered acceptable for a cleansing 30-day Paleo launch.*

Packable Paleo lunch

This idea comes from Melissa Joulwan, my coauthor of *Living Paleo For Dummies* (Wiley) and a recipe contributor for this book:

1. Place two servings of frozen vegetables in a portable container; drizzle olive oil over the top and add a generous sprinkle of garlic powder, salt, and ground black pepper.

2. Add a serving of protein on top — grilled chicken, frozen cooked shrimp, browned ground beef, or whatever you have on hand — and place the lid on the container.

3. In a separate container, place salad dressing or sauce.

4. When it's time to eat, warm the container of vegetables and protein. Transfer to a plate and drizzle with sauce.

Czech Meatballs

Prep time: 15 min • **Cook time:** 20–25 min • **Yield:** 6–8 servings

Ingredients	Directions
1 clove garlic, minced	**1** Preheat the oven to 400 degrees. Cover a large, rimmed baking sheet with parchment paper or aluminum foil.
½ tablespoon salt	
1 tablespoon caraway seeds	**2** In a large bowl, mix the garlic, salt, caraway, paprika, pepper, parsley, mustard, and egg with a fork until combined. With your hands, crumble the pork into the bowl and knead until all the ingredients are incorporated.
1 teaspoon ground paprika	
1 tablespoon pepper	
¼ cup minced fresh parsley	
1 tablespoon stone-ground mustard	**3** Moisten your hands with water and shake to remove excess. Measure a level tablespoon of pork and roll into a ball between your palms. Line up the meatballs on the prepared baking sheet about ½ inch apart.
1 egg	
2 pounds ground pork	
	4 Bake for 20 to 25 minutes until golden brown and cooked through.

Per serving: Calories 283 (From Fat 158); Fat 18g (Saturated 7g); Cholesterol 114mg; Sodium 540mg; Carbohydrate 1g (Dietary Fiber 0g); Protein 30g.

*Recipe courtesy Melissa Joulwan, author of Well Fed: Paleo Recipes for People Who Love to Eat and The Clothes Make the Girl (*www.theclothesmakethegirl.com*)*

*This recipe has been vetted by the team at Whole9 (*http://whole9life.com*) and is considered acceptable for a cleansing 30-day Paleo launch.*

Stuffed Bell Peppers

Prep time: 20 min • **Cook time:** 30 min • **Yield:** 4 servings

Ingredients	*Directions*
4 green bell peppers, tops removed and seeded	*1* Preheat the oven to 350 degrees.
3 tablespoons coconut oil, divided	*2* Wrap the green peppers in aluminum foil and place in a baking dish. Bake for 15 minutes; remove and set aside.
1 pound ground bison	
½ cup chopped onion	*3* In a skillet, heat 1 tablespoon of the coconut oil and cook the bison over medium heat until it's evenly brown. Remove to a separate bowl.
1 small zucchini, chopped	
½ a yellow bell pepper, chopped	
½ a red bell pepper, chopped	*4* Heat the remaining oil in the skillet and cook the onions, zucchini, and red and yellow bell peppers until tender. Add the spinach in the last 2 minutes to wilt.
1½ cups fresh spinach	
One 14.5-ounce can diced tomatoes	*5* Return the bison to the skillet. Mix in the tomatoes and the tomato paste and season with the Italian Seasoning. Add salt and pepper to taste.
1 tablespoon tomato paste	
1 teaspoon Italian Seasoning	*6* Stuff the green peppers with the bison mixture. Return the peppers to the oven and cook for another 15 minutes.
Salt and pepper to taste	

Per serving: Calories 350 (From Fat 182); Fat 20g (Saturated 13g); Cholesterol 80mg; Sodium 209mg; Carbohydrate 14g (Dietary Fiber 3g); Protein 32g.

Note: The recipe for Italian Seasoning is in Chapter 15.

Vary It! If you're unable to get ground bison, these peppers are just as delicious with ground beef.

Tip: These peppers are the perfect go-to lunch, so make plenty! They're easy to carry, easy to heat up, and perfectly balanced.

*This recipe has been vetted by the team at Whole9 (*http://whole9life.com*) and is considered acceptable for a cleansing 30-day Paleo launch.*

Chicken Club Wrap

Prep time: 5 min • **Yield:** 3 servings

Ingredients	*Directions*
3 large romaine lettuce leaves	*1* Wash the lettuce leaves and pat dry.
1 cup cooked chicken, diced	
½ a red bell pepper, diced	*2* In a small bowl, mix the remaining ingredients with a fork.
1 plum tomato, sliced	
½ an avocado, peeled, pitted, and diced	*3* Place the mixture into the center of the lettuce leaves. Wrap up and enjoy!
1 tablespoon Olive Oil Mayo	

Per serving: Calories 177 (From Fat 110); Fat 12g (Saturated 2g); Cholesterol 23mg; Sodium 220mg; Carbohydrate 10g (Dietary Fiber 3g); Protein 7g.

Note: Flip to Chapter 9 for the Olive Oil Mayo recipe.

Vary It! Add some chopped cooked bacon for extra smoky flavor and crunch.

*Recipe courtesy Mark Sisson, author of Primal Blueprint and Mark's Daily Apple (*www.marksdaily apple.com*)*

*This recipe has been vetted by the team at Whole9 (*http://whole9life.com*) and is considered acceptable for a cleansing 30-day Paleo launch.*

Kohlrabi Buffalo Wraps

Prep time: 10 min • **Cook time:** 10 min • **Yield:** 3 wraps

Ingredients	Directions
8 small or 3–4 large kohlrabies	**1** Cut the stems from the kohlrabies and then remove the leaves and set them aside; discard the stems. Bring a pot of water to a boil, add the leaves, and boil for 3 minutes. Drain in a colander and set aside.
2 teaspoons white wine vinegar	
1½ tablespoons macadamia nut oil	**2** Peel and grate the kohlrabies. In a bowl, whisk together the vinegar and macadamia nut oil with a pinch of salt and pepper. Drizzle over the grated kohlrabi. Set this slaw aside.
Pinch of salt and pepper, plus more to taste	
½ medium onion, diced	**3** Over medium heat, sauté the onion in the coconut oil until it's soft and just starting to brown.
1 teaspoon coconut oil	
¾ pound ground buffalo	**4** In a bowl, combine the buffalo, dill, parsley, paprika, and tomato paste. Add the buffalo mixture to the onion, breaking it up as it browns, about 5 minutes. Add salt and pepper to taste.
1½ tablespoons minced fresh dill	
1 tablespoon minced fresh parsley	
½ teaspoon sweet paprika	**5** To make a wrap, pile a spoonful of kohlrabi slaw and buffalo in the middle of a kohlrabi leaf and wrap the leaf around it.
1 teaspoon tomato paste	

Per serving: Calories 310 (From Fat 164); Fat 18g (Saturated 6g); Cholesterol 81mg; Sodium 121mg; Carbohydrate 8g (Dietary Fiber 4g); Protein 31g.

Note: If you never tried kohlrabi, this recipe is a great way to get your feet wet! Farmers' markets are a great way to score some of this Paleo-approved vegetable!

Recipe courtesy Mark Sisson, author of Primal Blueprint and Mark's Daily Apple (www.marksdaily apple.com)

This recipe has been vetted by the team at Whole9 (http://whole9life.com) and is considered acceptable for a cleansing 30-day Paleo launch.

Caveman Cobb Salad with Pan-Seared Tenderloin

Prep time: 15 min, plus roasting time • **Cook time:** 10 min • **Yield:** 2 servings

Ingredients	Directions
1 beet	**1** Preheat the oven to 350 degrees. Wrap the beet in foil and place it in a roasting pan. Peel the squash, remove the seeds, cube it, and place it in the pan with the beet.
1 small butternut squash	
One 8-ounce, 1-inch-thich beef tenderloin steak	
Kosher salt	**2** Roast for 45 to 60 minutes until a paring knife easily inserts all the way through the beet and squash cubes. Remove the pan from the oven and let cool for 10 minutes.
1 tablespoon olive oil	
3 cups spring mix	
2 hard-boiled eggs, quartered	**3** Remove the beet from the foil and peel it by hand. Slice the beet into thin strips and measure 1 cup of squash cubes. (Save the remaining roasted squash for another meal.)
12 cherry tomatoes, halved	
½ an avocado, peeled, pitted, and sliced	
Honey Pepper Vinaigrette to taste	**4** Heat a large sauté pan over high heat. Dry the beef on all sides with a paper towel and season one side with kosher salt.
	5 Add the olive oil to the preheated pan and place the steak in the pan, seasoned side down. Season the other side with kosher salt. Cook for approximately 2 minutes, or until you get a hard sear.
	6 Flip the steak and cook for another 60 to 90 seconds for medium-rare. (Adjust cooking times to achieve desired doneness.) Remove the steak from the pan and let it rest for 5 minutes before slicing against the grain.

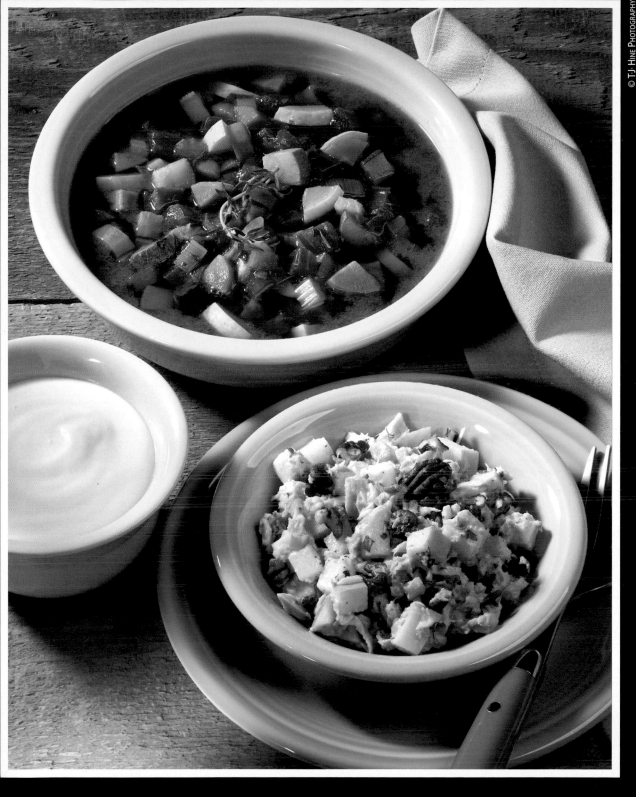

Who doesn't love a soup and salad combo for lunch or dinner? Pair the nutrient-dense Provençal Vegetable Soup (Chapter 7) with a Paleo-friendly Waldorf Tuna Salad (Chapter 8) made with creamy and delicious Olive Oil Mayo (Chapter 9).

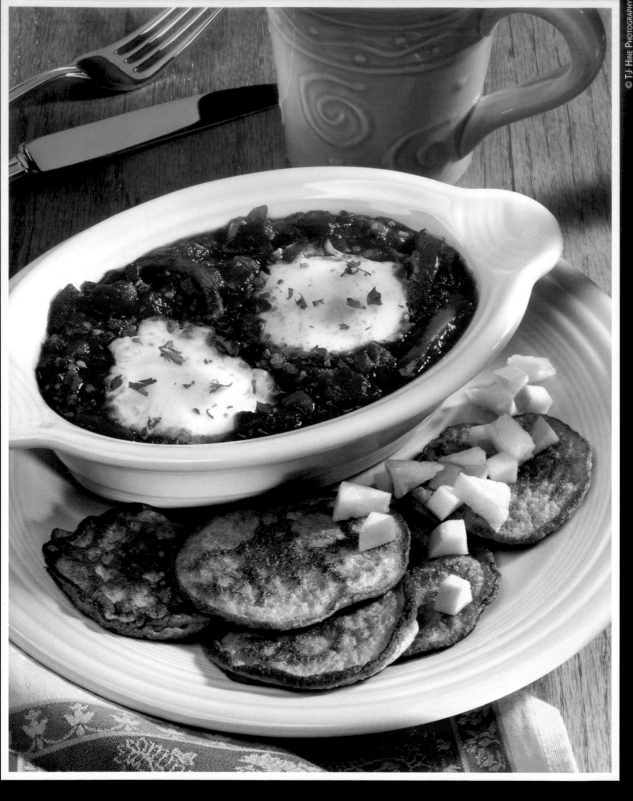

One important Paleo principle is to dial into how food makes you feel. Chapter 11 has numerous recipes to fuel you up for the day, including Mini Cinnamon Pancakes that your family will love and Eggs in Spicy Tomato Sauce that will keep you in the zone all morning.

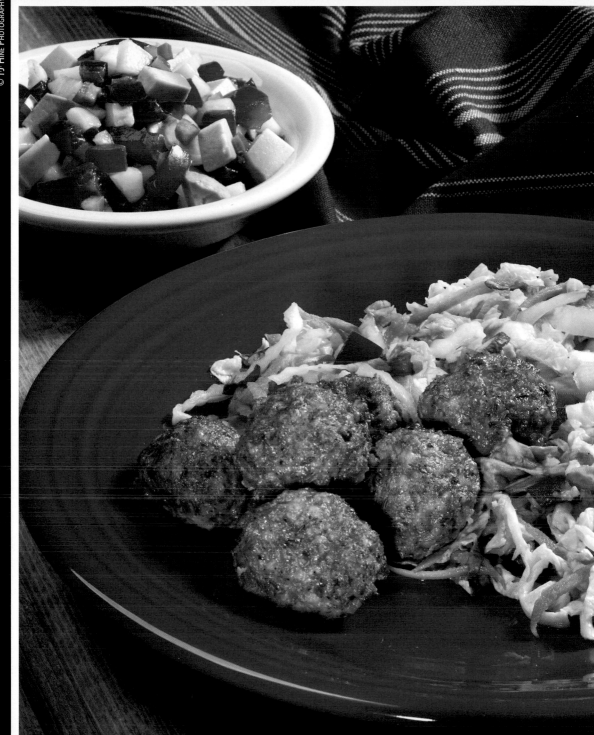

Try Paleo batch cooking each week to bring simplicity into your life. Easy make-ahead recipes such as Czech Meatballs (Chapter 12) and Cucumber Avocado Salsa (Chapter 9) are bursting with flavor. Kimchi (Chapter 16) is an Asian pickled condiment that really works at healing your intestines.

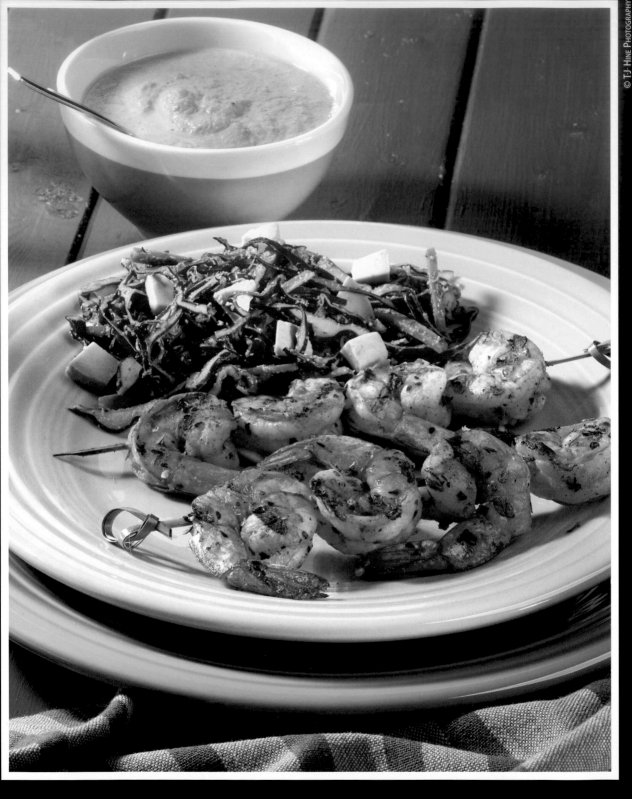

Introduce your family and friends to a Paleo-style cookout with the Grilled Buffalo Shrimp recipe in Chapter 13, with a side of Cabbage Slaw with Tangy Carrot Dressing from Chapter 12. It won't be long before they return the invitation and host their own Paleo cookout!

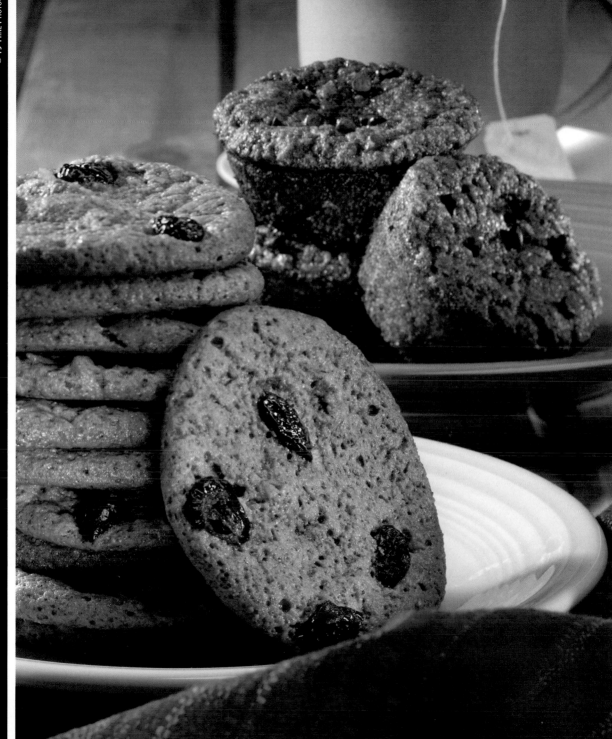

If you think that Paleo cooking means saying goodbye to gooey, delicious desserts and sweet treats, you'll be happy to discover many Paleo-friendly dessert recipes in Chapter 17, including Cranberry Ginger Cookies and Banana Cacao Muffins.

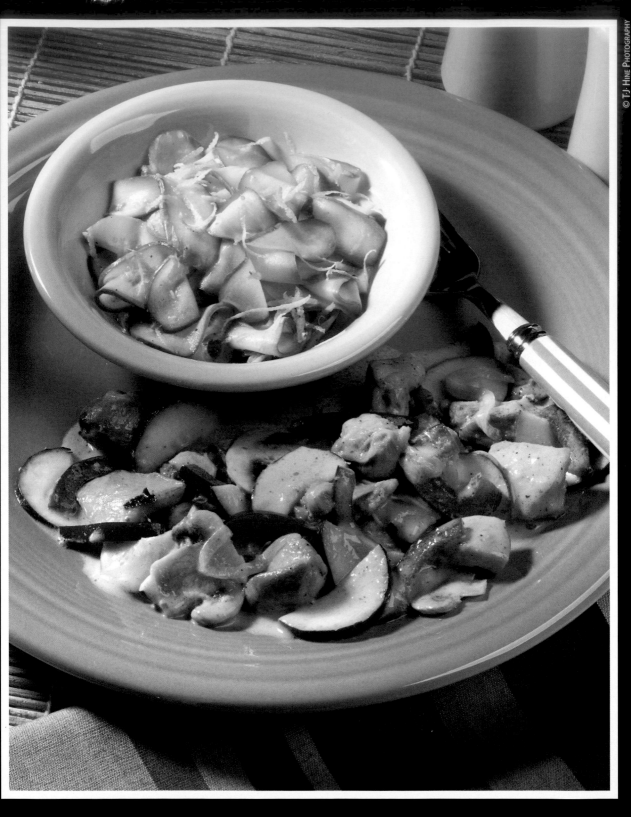

The Paleo diet is loaded with protein and vegetables. You get both — plus tons of flavor and spice — with the Thai Green Curry Chicken (Chapter 14) and Lemon Cucumber Noodles with Cumin (Chapter 16). The international flair of these dishes will warm your spirit and tantalize your taste buds.

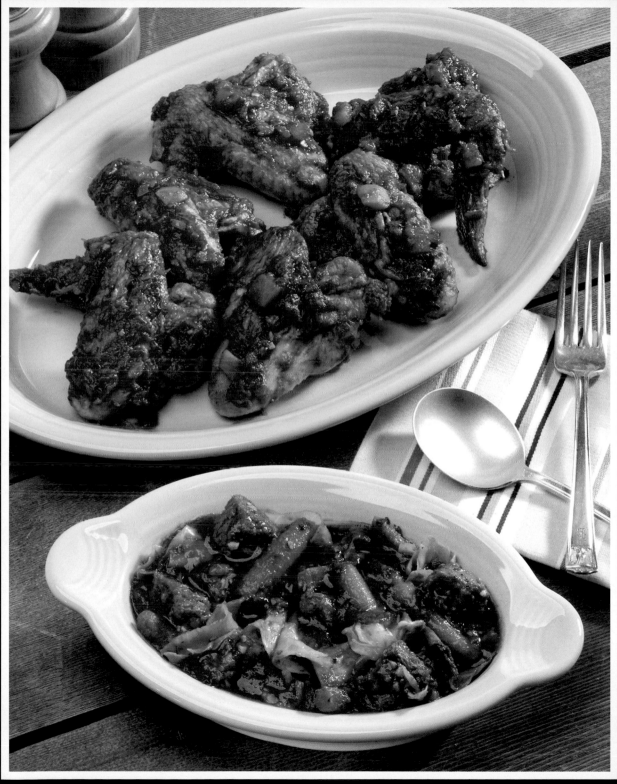

Making meals using a slow cooker is both convenient and wholesome. Whip up the Pineapple and Mango Sweet Heat Chicken Wings to feed a crowd, or fix the Cheater Pork Stew before work and come home to a dinner that's ready to eat. You can find these and other slow cooker recipes in Chapter 18.

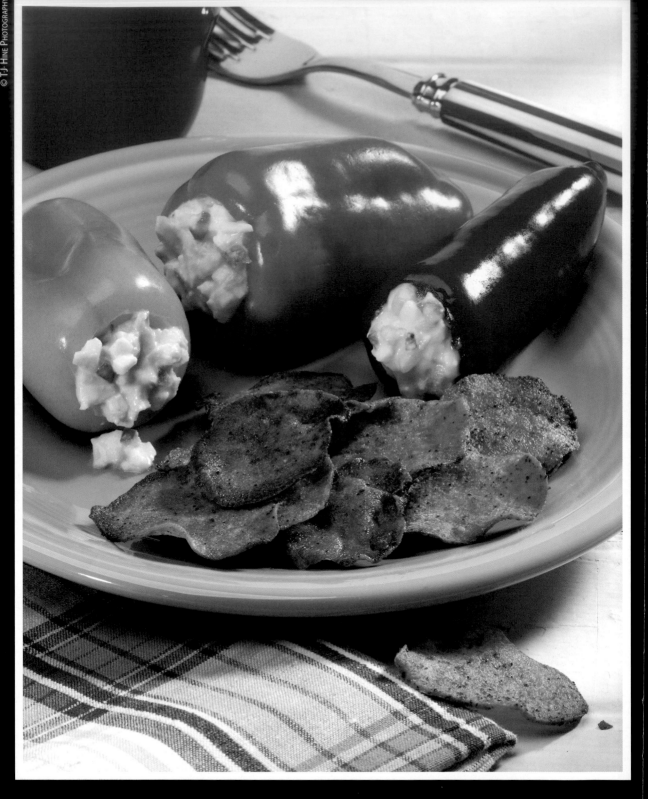

Teach children about nutrition and healthier foods at a young age, and you'll see lasting effects. The recipes in Chapter 19, like Lunchbox Stuffed Peppers, are proven kid favorites. Pair them with some Sweet Potato Chips (Chapter 10), and your kids will be begging for more Paleo goodies.

7   Place the spring mix in the center of a large plate.

8   Mentally divide the plate into 5 segments and then place the eggs, beets, squash, tomatoes, and avocado in separate sections. Dress the salad with Honey Pepper Vinaigrette to taste. Top with sliced beef tenderloin and enjoy!

Per serving: Calories 514 (From Fat 243); Fat 27g (Saturated 9g); Cholesterol 275mg; Sodium 439mg; Carbohydrate 20g (Dietary Fiber 8g); Protein 46g.

Note: Look for the Honey Pepper Vinaigrette in Chapter 9.

Tip: When peeling the roasted beet, wear latex gloves to prevent your hands from turning purple.

Recipe courtesy Nick Massie, chef and author of Paleo Nick (`http://paleonick.com`*)*

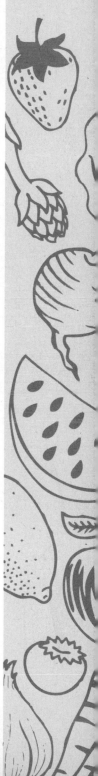

Beef and Broccoli with Roasted Sweet Potatoes

Prep time: 10 min • **Cook time:** 40 min • **Yield:** 4 servings

Ingredients	Directions
2 large sweet potatoes, peeled and chopped into ½-inch cubes	*1* Preheat the oven to 375 degrees.
2 tablespoons olive oil	*2* In a large bowl, combine the sweet potatoes, olive oil, garlic powder, and cinnamon (if desired). Mix well so that the potatoes are completely covered in oil and spices.
¼ teaspoon garlic powder	
½ teaspoon ground cinnamon (optional)	*3* Place the potatoes in a 9-x-13-inch baking dish and arrange in a single layer. Bake for 30 minutes, turning the mixture once. Remove from the oven and set aside.
1 tablespoon plus 1 teaspoon coconut oil, divided	*4* Heat 1 tablespoon of the coconut oil in a large skillet until it's liquid and shimmering. Add the garlic, onion, salt, pepper, and chili powder. Cook until the onions are soft.
3 cloves garlic, minced	
1 medium onion, chopped	*5* Add the beef to the onions and garlic, breaking up the beef as it browns. Drain the excess fat; remove the beef from the skillet and set aside.
½ teaspoon salt	
½ teaspoon pepper	*6* Add the remaining coconut oil to the skillet and heat until the oil is liquid and shimmering. Add the broccoli to pan and cook until it's bright green.
½ teaspoon chili powder	
1 pound ground beef	
2 cups chopped broccoli	*7* Add the cooked beef and the sweet potatoes to the broccoli, mix well, and heat through. Serve immediately.

Per serving: Calories 489 (From Fat 288); Fat 32g (Saturated 13g); Cholesterol 100mg; Sodium 466mg; Carbohydrate 19g (Dietary Fiber 4g); Protein 32g.

Tip: You can roast the sweet potatoes the day before.

Tip: This recipe is a great recovery food after a Paleo workout! Make this delicious meal in bulk.

This recipe has been vetted by the team at Whole9 (http://whole9life.com) and is considered acceptable for a cleansing 30-day Paleo launch.

Chapter 13

Paleo Seafood and Fishmonger Meals

In This Chapter

▶ Getting the best seafood products

▶ Discovering fantastic Paleo fish and shellfish meals

You know that great warm feeling you get when you think of summertime vacations spent by the shore? There's something about seafood, like a plate of Creamy Baked Scallops, that can bring you back to the seaside with just one whiff. You instantly feel lighter and more relaxed.

I've dedicated this chapter to all those summer traditions and meals you enjoy — and to the people you love to share them with. In addition to all the recipes in this chapter, you can find a recipe for Dilly Chili Roasted King Salmon, among others, online at www.dummies.com/extras/paleo cookbook.

If you're a vegetarian who eats fish and seafood, you can enjoy all the recipes in this chapter except for the Garlic Shrimp Scampi, Scallops with Bacon, and Roasted Oysters.

Buying Fresh Fish

Some people buy only frozen fish and seafood or avoid these versatile and nutritious protein sources altogether because they aren't sure how to buy quality fresh items. Here are some tips to help you enjoy the healthiest, freshest fish and seafood possible:

- Go to only the best fishmongers or to a reputable store and ask for the catch of the day. The fish store or counter should never smell fishy or like you're standing in the middle of a low tide.

- Fish should have a salty air scent, not a fishy smell.

- Fish should be firm, shiny, and bounce back when you touch it.

- Fish fillets should be moist, and the flesh shouldn't separate or be discolored. Gaps in the meat as well as brown or yellow edges are signs of aging.

- Fish shouldn't have liquid on the meat. That milky look on fish means the fish is aging.

- Whole fish should have bright, clear (not cloudy) eyes, and bright red gills.

- Shrimp should be firm and moist with translucent shells.

- Clams, mussels, and oysters should have tightly closed shells. If the shells gape slightly, tap them with a knife. If they don't close, discard them.

- Shucked clams, mussels, and oysters should be plump. Make sure their liquid is clear and slightly opalescent.

You don't want *frankenfish* — fish loaded with bad stuff like toxins such as mercury, PCBs, and hormones or antibiotics that you ingest when you eat the fish. Two great resources that can help guide you to the best choices in your area are www.montereybayaquarium.org/cr/seafoodwatch.aspx and www.cleanfish.com. Wild-caught, fresh fish is always best!

Fish is filled with omega-3 fatty acids, which are critical to the function of every cell in your body. Unfortunately, most people are deficient in these crucial fatty acids, so finding a clean source of fish or taking purified fish oil or a fish oil tablet to help bump up your levels is worthwhile.

Grilled Buffalo Shrimp

Prep time: 5 min • **Cook time:** 6–8 min • **Yield:** 4 servings

Ingredients	*Directions*
1 clove garlic, minced	**1** Combine all the ingredients except the shrimp in a bowl and mix well. Add the shrimp and mix well, ensuring an even coating.
¼ cup hot sauce	
1 teaspoon coconut oil, melted	
1 teaspoon crushed red pepper	**2** Grease the grill with coconut oil spray or a little extra melted coconut oil. Preheat your grill to about 400 degrees. Use a grill rack if you have it so your shrimp don't fall through the grates; preheat the rack on the grill. If you don't have a rack, arrange the shrimp on skewers.
1 teaspoon Italian seasoning	
¼ teaspoon cayenne pepper	
¼ teaspoon Celtic sea salt	
¼ teaspoon pepper	
24 medium shrimp, peeled and deveined	**3** When your grill is heated, place the shrimp on the grill and close the lid. Allow to cook for 1 to 2 minutes, and then flip and finish cooking for 1 to 2 minutes on the other side.
	4 Serve and enjoy.

Per serving: Calories 43 (From Fat 15); Fat 1.5g (Saturated 1g); Cholesterol 53mg; Sodium 690mg; Carbohydrate 1g (Dietary Fiber 0g); Protein 6g.

Tip: If you have time, let the shrimp marinate in the fridge for 30 minutes or so before moving to Step 2. If you use skewers, double skewer the shrimp — use two parallel skewers — to prevent the shrimp from twisting around the skewers as you flip them over. You can broil the shrimp if you don't have an outdoor grill or if the temperature outside is too cold to use one.

*Recipe courtesy George Bryant, CEO and author of Civilized Caveman Cooking Creations (*http://civilizedcavemancooking.com*)*

*This recipe has been vetted by the team at Whole9 (*http://whole9life.com*) and is considered acceptable for a cleansing 30-day Paleo launch.*

Coconut Shrimp with Sweet and Spicy Sauce

Prep time: 10 min • **Cook time:** 5 min • **Yield:** 2 servings

Ingredients	Directions
1 cup chopped fresh pineapple	*1* Preheat the oven to 450 degrees. Line a baking sheet with aluminum foil, shiny side down.
1 jalapeño, seeded (optional) and chopped	*2* Blend the pineapple, jalapeño, lime juice, and onions in a blender or food processor on high until the consistency of the sauce is smooth with small bits. Set this sauce aside.
Juice of 1 lime	
¼ medium white or red onion, chopped	
½ cup almond flour	*3* In a gallon-size zip-top bag, combine the almond flour, coconut, garlic, cumin, salt, and pepper. Beat the egg white in a small bowl.
½ cup unsweetened shredded coconut	
1 clove garlic, minced	*4* Coat the shrimp generously in the egg wash and then place them in the zip-top bag. Shake the bag so that all the shrimp are evenly coated with the breading mixture.
½ teaspoon ground cumin	
¼ teaspoon salt	
¼ teaspoon pepper	*5* Remove the shrimp from the bag and place on the baking sheet. Bake for 2 minutes on the middle rack of your oven. Flip the shrimp over and bake for 3 minutes.
1 egg white	
12 large shrimp, peeled, deveined, and butterflied	*6* Remove from the oven and serve with the sauce for dipping.

Per serving: Calories 451 (From Fat 206); Fat 23g (Saturated 7g); Cholesterol 214mg; Sodium 1,290mg; Carbohydrate 32g (Dietary Fiber 7g); Protein 33g.

Note: Leaving the seeds in the jalapeño will make the sauce spicier.

Tip: You can use this dipping sauce on all kinds of food. Try it on eggs or chicken for a delicious twist.

*Recipe courtesy George Bryant, CEO and author of Civilized Caveman Cooking Creations (*http://civilizedcavemancooking.com*)*

*This recipe has been vetted by the team at Whole9 (*http://whole9life.com*) and is considered acceptable for a cleansing 30-day Paleo launch.*

Garlic Shrimp Scampi

Prep time: 10 min • **Cook time:** 40–60 min • **Yield:** 4 servings

Ingredients	*Directions*
1 medium spaghetti squash	*1* Preheat the oven 375 degrees. Line a baking sheet with parchment paper.
½ medium red onion, diced	
3 cloves garlic, minced	*2* Cut the squash in half lengthwise and scrape out the seeds. Place the squash cut side down on the baking sheet and sprinkle the parchment around it with water. Cook for 30 to 40 minutes until tender but not mushy.
¼ cup melted ghee	
1 tablespoon chopped fresh parsley	
Pinch of salt	
Pinch of pepper	*3* Remove the squash from the oven and let it cool for 5 minutes. Shred the flesh with a fork to make spaghetti.
½ cup chicken broth	
1 pound medium shrimp, peeled and deveined	*4* Reset the oven temperature to broil. Place the onion, garlic, ghee, and parsley in the bottom of a 9-x-13-inch baking dish. Add the salt and pepper and pour the chicken broth over everything.
1 lemon, quartered	
	5 Broil the onion mixture on the middle oven rack for 5 minutes. Add the shrimp and broil for another 5 minutes, flipping the shrimp halfway through.
	6 Arrange the squash on the plate and top with the shrimp mixture. Sprinkle with freshly squeezed lemon juice.

Per serving: Calories 151 (From Fat 27); Fat 3g (Saturated 1g); Cholesterol 290mg; Sodium 999mg; Carbohydrate 7g (Dietary Fiber 2g); Protein 25g.

Note: You can find a recipe for ghee in Chapter 9.

*Recipe courtesy George Bryant, CEO and author of Civilized Caveman Cooking Creations (*http://civilizedcavemancooking.com*)*

*This recipe has been vetted by the team at Whole9 (*http://whole9life.com*) and is considered acceptable for a cleansing 30-day Paleo launch.*

Creamy Baked Scallops

Prep time: 10 min • **Cook time:** 10 min • **Yield:** 2 servings

Ingredients	Directions
12 medium sea scallops	**1** Preheat the oven to 475 degrees.
1 cup chopped red onion	**2** Evenly space the scallops in the bottom of an 8-x-8-inch baking dish.
1 teaspoon coconut oil	
3 cloves garlic, minced	**3** In a large skillet, sauté the onions over medium-high heat in the coconut oil until they start to turn opaque.
½ cup tomato sauce	
¼ cup coconut milk	**4** Lower the heat to medium-low. Add the garlic, tomato sauce, coconut milk, oregano, salt, and pepper, and mix well. Pour the mixture over the scallops in the baking dish. Cover with the chopped tomatoes.
¼ teaspoon dried oregano	
¼ teaspoon salt	
¼ teaspoon pepper	
1 cup diced tomatoes	**5** Bake 10 to 15 minutes until the tomatoes start to brown and the sauce is bubbling.
	6 Remove from the oven and serve in a bowl with plenty of sauce.

Per serving: Calories 367 (From Fat 107); Fat 12g (Saturated 8g); Cholesterol 70mg; Sodium 1,942mg; Carbohydrate 28g (Dietary Fiber 3.5g); Protein 39g.

Tip: Any tomato sauce you have in your pantry works for this dish. Just be sure it's unsweetened.

Recipe courtesy George Bryant, CEO and author of Civilized Caveman Cooking Creations (http://civilizedcavemancooking.com)

This recipe has been vetted by the team at Whole9 (http://whole9life.com) and is considered acceptable for a cleansing 30-day Paleo launch.

Scallops with Bacon

Prep time: 5 min • **Cook time:** 4 min • **Yield:** 2 servings

Ingredients	Directions
1 ounce uncured, nitrate-free, no-sugar-added bacon 2 tablespoons lime juice 2 tablespoons coconut oil, divided 6 fresh sea scallops Sprinkle of Celtic sea salt Sprinkle of pepper 1 tablespoon chopped fresh tarragon	**1** Slice the bacon crosswise into thin pieces and cook in a skillet over medium-high heat until crisp but not dry. Transfer the bacon to a paper towel or dish. **2** In a small bowl, combine the lime juice and 1 tablespoon of the coconut oil. Coat the scallops in the oil mixture and sprinkle with salt and pepper. **3** Sear the scallops in a skillet over medium-high heat for about 1½ minutes, flip them, and sear the other side for another 1½ minutes until they're opaque and glossy. Transfer them to a separate plate. **4** Reduce the heat to medium. Add the remaining lime juice to the skillet and begin scraping the brown bits from the bottom of the pan. **5** Add 2 tablespoons of water, the bacon, and the scallops (in that order). Stir to blend the juices; cook 1 minute to allow the flavors to combine. **6** Serve the scallops with the bacon and pan juices. Sprinkle with the tarragon.

Per serving: Calories 295 (From Fat 180); Fat 20g (Saturated 14g); Cholesterol 50mg; Sodium 896mg; Carbohydrate 7g (Dietary Fiber 0g); Protein 23g.

Note: Pair this delicious dish with Kale with a Kick Salad (Chapter 8), Simple Sautéed Kohlrabi (Chapter 16), or Brussels Sprouts with Cranberries and Almonds (Chapter 16).

*Recipe courtesy Mark Sisson, author of Primal Blueprint and Mark's Daily Apple (*www.marksdaily apple.com*)*

*This recipe has been vetted by the team at Whole9 (*http://whole9life.com*) and is considered acceptable for a cleansing 30-day Paleo launch.*

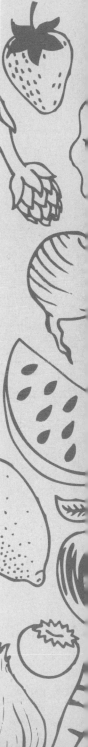

Roasted Oysters

Prep time: 15 min • **Cook time:** 25 min • **Yield:** 6 servings

Ingredients	Directions
5 ounces frozen spinach	*1* Preheat the oven to 450 degrees. Prepare the spinach according to the package instructions.
12 oysters	
4 tablespoons olive oil, divided	*2* Shuck the oysters and release the meat from the cup portion of the shell; be careful to retain the liquor, or juice, in the oyster shell.
½ cup minced garlic	
½ cup minced shallots	*3* Press the shucked oysters securely into bed of foil on a baking sheet so as to not spill any juice.
1 bell pepper, seeded and finely diced	
Kosher salt and pepper to taste	*4* Preheat a large skillet over high heat. Add 2 tablespoons of the olive oil, the garlic, and the shallots and sauté for 2 minutes. Add the bell pepper and cooked spinach; mix well, breaking up the spinach. Cook for another 2 minutes.
Chili powder to taste	
Juice of ¼ lemon	
2 slices prosciutto, each cut into six pieces	*5* Season with salt, pepper, and chili powder to taste. Stir in the lemon juice and remove the skillet from the heat.
	6 Spoon the vegetable mixture into the oyster cups. Top each oyster with a piece of prosciutto and then the place pan on the bottom rack of the oven.
	7 Bake for 7 minutes and then transfer to the top rack of the oven. Reset the oven temperature to broil to finish cooking and crisp up the prosciutto.
	8 Remove the oysters from oven, drizzle lightly with the remaining olive oil, and allow to rest for a few minutes before serving.

Per serving: Calories 146 (From Fat 96); Fat 11g (Saturated 2g); Cholesterol 20mg; Sodium 227mg; Carbohydrate 11g (Dietary Fiber 1g); Protein 5g.

Vary It! Be creative with this recipe. You can substitute partially cooked bacon for the prosciutto; add fresh herbs to the veggie mixture; or garnish with fresh herbs, lemon zest, lobster claws, or a slice of delicately seared sea scallop. Just be sure to keep added seafood in the shellfish family.

*Recipe courtesy Nick Massie, chef and author of Paleo Nick (*http://paleonick.com*)*

*This recipe has been vetted by the team at Whole9 (*http://whole9life.com*) and is considered acceptable for a cleansing 30-day Paleo launch.*

Macadamia Nut Crusted Mahi-Mahi

Prep time: 10 min, plus marinating time • **Cook time:** 10 min • **Yield:** 2 servings

Ingredients	Directions
Two 6- to 8-ounce mahi-mahi fillets **1 cup coconut milk** **¼ cup roasted macadamia nuts** **1 tablespoon coconut flour** **1 tablespoon almond flour** **2 tablespoons coconut oil, melted and divided** **Pinch of salt** **Pinch of pepper** **½ cup shredded unsweetened coconut**	*1* Place the fillets in a zip-top bag with the coconut milk and let sit at room temperature for 30 to 60 minutes. *2* Preheat the oven to 425 degrees. *3* Grind the macadamia nuts in a blender or food processor until they're coarsely ground. Add the coconut flour and almond flour and process further to mix well. Transfer the nut mixture to a bowl. *4* Add 1 tablespoon of melted coconut oil to the nut mixture and mix well. *5* Line a baking sheet with aluminum foil and brush with the remaining coconut oil so your fish doesn't stick. Place the fillets on the baking sheet and salt and pepper each side of the fish to your liking. *6* Bake the fish for 5 minutes and then remove it from the oven. Flip the fillets over and spread the nut mixture over them, pressing it down so it sticks. Sprinkle the shredded coconut on top to your liking. *7* Bake for an additional 8 to 10 minutes or until the coconut and macadamia nuts are nicely browned. *8* Remove from the oven and let sit for 10 minutes before serving.

Per serving: Calories 781 (From Fat 585); Fat 65g (Saturated 45g); Cholesterol 146mg; Sodium 488mg; Carbohydrate 15g (Dietary Fiber 8g); Protein 42g.

Tip: Serve this dish with fresh pineapple for an absolutely delicious meal.

Recipe courtesy George Bryant, CEO and author of Civilized Caveman Cooking Creations (`http://civilizedcavemancooking.com`*)*

This recipe has been vetted by the team at Whole9 (`http://whole9life.com`*) and is considered acceptable for a cleansing 30-day Paleo launch.*

Olive-Oil Braised Albacore

Prep time: 10 min • **Cook time:** 30 min • **Yield:** 4 servings

Ingredients	Directions
2 pounds skinless fresh albacore fillet	**1** Preheat the oven to 350 degrees.
Pinch of kosher salt	
Pinch of pepper	**2** Cut the albacore crosswise into 1½-inch steaks. Season both sides with salt and pepper.
4 cloves garlic, roughly chopped	**3** Place the steaks in a single layer in a casserole dish and top with the garlic. Pour the olive oil in the dish until it reaches halfway up the sides of the fish. (Use more or less oil as needed.)
⅔ cup extra-virgin olive oil	
1 medium lemon, quartered	
	4 Cover the dish with foil and bake for 10 minutes. Carefully flip the fish and bake for another 10 minutes, covered. The albacore is finished when it's barely cooked through.
	5 Let the tuna cool to room temperature and serve with the olive-oil braising liquid and a squeeze of lemon juice.

Per serving: Calories 610 (From Fat 372); Fat 41g (Saturated 5g); Cholesterol 100mg; Sodium 771mg; Carbohydrate 4g (Dietary Fiber 1.5g); Protein 65g.

Tip: This dish stores well in the fridge. Just keep the fish in the olive-oil braising liquid and you'll have emergency protein ready to eat.

Note: You can pair this dish nicely with the delicious salads in Chapter 8. You can also turn to a vegetarian side, such as the Italian Broccoli or the Cocoa Cauliflower in Chapter 16.

*Recipe courtesy Michelle Tam, author of Nom Nom Paleo (*http://nomnompaleo.com*)*

*This recipe has been vetted by the team at Whole9 (*http://whole9life.com*) and is considered acceptable for a cleansing 30-day Paleo launch.*

Salmon a L'Afrique du Nord

Prep time: 5 min, plus marinating time • **Cook time:** 6–7 min • **Yield:** 8 servings

Ingredients	Directions
1 tablespoon coconut oil, melted	**1** Mix the coconut oil, orange juice, ginger, cumin, coriander, paprika, salt, and cayenne in a small bowl to form a paste the consistency of thick salad dressing.
1 tablespoon fresh orange juice	
1½ teaspoons dried ginger	**2** Place the salmon in a glass baking dish and massage the marinade over the salmon. Cover and refrigerate for 30 minutes.
1½ teaspoons ground cumin	
1½ teaspoons ground coriander	**3** Preheat a gas grill on high with the lid closed for about 10 minutes.
½ teaspoon paprika	
1½ teaspoons salt	**4** Place the salmon skin-side down on the grill, close the lid, and cook for 3 minutes. Check the salmon; the skin should be a little blackened and starting to separate from the pink flesh.
¼ teaspoon ground cayenne pepper	
1½ pounds skin-on salmon fillets	**5** Flip the salmon, close the lid, and cook an additional 3 minutes. Serve immediately.

Per serving: Calories 169 (From Fat 97); Fat 11g (Saturated 3g); Cholesterol 49mg; Sodium 485mg; Carbohydrate 1g (Dietary Fiber 0g); Protein 17g.

*Recipe courtesy Melissa Joulwan, author of Well Fed: Paleo Recipes for People Who Love to Eat and The Clothes Make the Girl (*www.theclothesmakethegirl.com*)*

*This recipe has been vetted by the team at Whole9 (*http://whole9life.com*) and is considered acceptable for a cleansing 30-day Paleo launch.*

Chapter 14

Protein Recipes for Paleo Meat-Lovers

- -

In This Chapter

▶ Understanding that not all meats are created equal

▶ Trying out amazing pork, chicken, lamb, and beef dishes

- -

*P*aleo protein has a certain punch. It's nutritionally dense food that provides you with what you need to build a healthy body. To keep yourself healthy and satisfied, you can enjoy any protein dish any time of day and for any meal of the day.

This chapter is loaded with a variety of protein recipes that feature pork, chicken, lamb, and beef. All the proteins in this chapter are snuggled up with other yummy ingredients — like broccoli, bell peppers, olives, tomatoes, sweet potatoes, ginger, and even chocolate — that make them really pop.

If you're looking for a fantastic dinner, try some outrageously delicious, award-winning Chocolate Chili. Maybe you want to be adventurous and try some Thai Green Curry Chicken. How about some Sausage and Spinach Stuffed Portobello Mushrooms for breakfast or some Tandoori Chicken Thighs for lunch? Or head to www.dummies.com/extras/paleocookbook for more great recipes, including Chicken Wings with Pineapple and Poblanos and Oven-Braised Mexican Beef.

Shopping for Top-Quality Meats

Health is contagious. The healthier the food, the more health it brings to your body. Of course, the opposite is true as well. You may have heard some of the debate over grass-fed and grain-fed meats; the animals' diet is one factor that makes a big difference in the meat you eat. One of the biggest differences between grass-fed and grain-fed animals is the overall fat content. Take beef, for example. Grass-fed beef is lower in total fat and omega-6 fatty acids. The opposite is true of grain-fed animals. A healthy diet has an omega-6 fatty acid to omega-3 fatty acid ratio of about 4:1. The ratio of omega-6s to omega-3s in grass-fed animals is about 3:1. Grain-fed beef ratios exceed 20:1 omega-6s to omega-3s.

When you're deciding where to spend your money at the grocery store, keep the following facts in mind to help you make the best choice in regard to meat quality:

- Animals that are pasture raised and forage on the natural diet of grass have less stress and live healthier lives. There's little or no need to treat them with antibiotics or drugs.

- Grass-fed meat is a great source of *conjugated linoleic acid* (CLA), which is a good component in fat found primarily in the meat and dairy products from *ruminant* (cud-chewing) animals. It reduces the risk of heart disease, cancer, obesity, and diabetes and boosts immunity. Grain-fed animals tend to be lower in CLA than their grass-eating relatives.

- Grass-fed meat is higher in B vitamins, calcium, magnesium, and potassium than meat from grain-fed animals.

- Meat from grass-fed cattle typically has a much lower risk of E. coli because the cows are cleaner at the time of slaughter and are typically processed by a skilled local butcher or farmer who ensures the meat doesn't come in contact with feces.

- Grass-fed beef has ten times the amount of vitamin A and three times more vitamin E than grain-fed beef. It's also safe from mad cow disease (MCD).

- Pasture-raised, locally sourced poultry is the cleanest source of chicken and turkey you can purchase. The birds are able to roam freely in their environment, where they eat bugs, nutritious grasses, and other plants that are a part of their natural diet. Organic, free-range poultry is also a good choice. Birds consume organic feed and have access to the outdoors. They are not given antibiotics unless they are ill.

If you're going to eat pork, make sure it comes from an organic, pasture-raised source. Otherwise, it's just too unhealthy; you're simply better off choosing another protein source. When selecting deli meats, make sure they're organic, gluten-free, and nitrite-free.

Winter Squash and Sausage Hash

Prep time: 15 min • **Cook time:** 25 min • **Yield:** 2 servings

Ingredients	*Directions*
2 cups ½-inch-diced winter squash	*1* Preheat the oven to 375 degrees.
1 cup diced mushrooms	*2* In a medium bowl, toss the squash, mushrooms, garlic, and sausage together.
2 cloves garlic, crushed	
½ pound spicy sausage (no-sugar added), casing removed and meat diced into 1-inch cubes	*3* Spread the vegetable mixture into a baking dish, making sure not to overcrowd, and bake for 25 minutes or until the veggies are tender and the sausage is browned.
1 tablespoon coconut oil	
4 eggs	*4* While the veggie mixture is baking, heat a medium skillet over medium heat. Starting with half the oil and adding more as needed, fry the eggs, two at a time, to your desired doneness.
Salt and pepper to taste	
Fresh parsley for garnish	
	5 Remove the vegetable mixture from the oven and top with the fried eggs. Garnish with parsley and salt and pepper to taste.

Per serving: Calories 476 (From Fat 272); Fat 30g (Saturated 13g); Cholesterol 455mg; Sodium 1,167mg; Carbohydrate 18g (Dietary Fiber 4g); Protein 35g.

Recipe courtesy Arsy Vartanian, author of Rubies & Radishes (www.rubiesandradishes.com)

This recipe has been vetted by the team at Whole9 (http://whole9life.com) and is considered acceptable for a cleansing 30-day Paleo launch.

Sausage and Spinach Stuffed Portobello Mushrooms

Prep time: 10 min • **Cook time:** 30 min • **Yield:** 4 servings

Ingredients	Directions
4 large cap portobello mushrooms	*1* Preheat the oven to 400 degrees with the rack in the center of the oven. Place a foil-lined baking sheet in the oven.
¼ cup plus 2 tablespoons melted ghee, divided	
Kosher salt	*2* Wipe the tops of the mushrooms with a damp cloth and scoop out the gills and stems with a spoon. Use a sharp paring knife to cut a shallow *X* on the top of each mushroom cap.
Pepper	
½ a small onion, minced	
1 pound bulk sausage (no-sugar-added)	*3* Brush the mushrooms all over with ¼ cup of the ghee and season with salt and pepper.
2 cups marinara sauce	
1 large egg, lightly beaten	*4* Place the mushrooms on the hot baking sheet, top side down. Bake for 10 minutes; flip the mushrooms over and bake for another 10 minutes.
10 ounces frozen spinach, defrosted and squeezed dry	
1 tablespoon coconut flour	*5* Remove the tray from the oven and let the mushrooms cool to room temperature. Increase the oven temperature to broil.

6 While the mushrooms are roasting, heat the remaining ghee in a large skillet over medium heat. Sauté the onions with salt and pepper until they're soft and translucent.

7 Add the sausage to the skillet, breaking it up with a wooden spoon. Cook the meat until it's no longer pink. Drain all the fat and remove the filling to a medium bowl; let it cool to room temperature.

8 Warm the marinara sauce in a small saucepan over low heat. When the sausage filling is cool, add the egg, spinach, and coconut flour and pinch of salt and pepper. Mix to combine.

9 Clean the mushroom liquid off the original baking sheet and replace the mushrooms on the sheet. Pile the stuffing onto each cap, pressing down to make the stuffing compact.

10 Place the tray under the broiler for about 5 minutes, rotating halfway through the cooking time. Remove the mushrooms from the oven when the stuffing is evenly browned.

11 Top the baked mushrooms with the heated marinara sauce and serve immediately.

Per serving: Calories 639 (From Fat 474); Fat 52g (Saturated 18g); Cholesterol 131mg; Sodium 1,911mg; Carbohydrate 21g (Dietary Fiber 6g); Protein 23g.

Note: You can find a ghee recipe in Chapter 9.

*Recipe courtesy Michelle Tam, author of Nom Nom Paleo (*http://nomnompaleo.com*)*

*This recipe has been vetted by the team at Whole9 (*http://whole9life.com*) and is considered acceptable for a cleansing 30-day Paleo launch.*

Citrus Carnitas

Prep time: 5 min • **Cook time:** 2–3 hr • **Yield:** 8 servings

Ingredients

1 tablespoon ground cumin

1 tablespoon garlic powder

½ tablespoon salt

1 teaspoon ground coriander

1 teaspoon pepper

¼–1 teaspoon ground cayenne pepper to taste

3 pounds boneless pork shoulder

½ cup lime juice

½ cup lemon juice

1 tablespoon coconut oil

Directions

1 In a large zip-top bag, combine the cumin, garlic powder, salt, coriander, black pepper, and cayenne; shake to mix well.

2 With a sharp knife, trim the excess fat off the pork shoulder and cut the pork into large chunks. Place the pork in the bag and shake until it's coated with the spices.

3 Transfer the pork to a large stockpot. Add the lime and lemon juices and then add enough water to just cover the meat.

4 Bring the pot to a rapid boil over high heat; reduce the heat to keep a steady, strong simmer with the pot uncovered. (Turn on the exhaust fan over your stovetop for this step.)

5 After 2 hours, check the pot. The water level should be much lower and maybe even almost gone.

6 Heat a large skillet with the coconut oil over medium-high heat and carefully transfer the pork to the skillet. Brown the pork on all sides.

7 Transfer the pork to a plate and let it rest for 5 minutes before serving.

Per serving: Calories 283 (From Fat 135); Fat 15g (Saturated 4.5g); Cholesterol 124mg; Sodium 1,967mg; Carbohydrate 4g (Dietary Fiber 0.5g); Protein 33g.

Recipe courtesy Melissa Joulwan, author of Well Fed: Paleo Recipes for People Who Love to Eat and The Clothes Make the Girl (www.theclothesmakethegirl.com)

This recipe has been vetted by the team at Whole9 (http://whole9life.com) and is considered acceptable for a cleansing 30-day Paleo launch.

Thai Green Curry Chicken

Prep time: 5 min • **Cook time:** 15 min • **Yield:** 4 servings

Ingredients	*Directions*
3-inch piece of lemongrass	*1* Thinly slice the pale yellow portion of the lemongrass and process it in a blender or small food chopper or processor.
2 tablespoons coconut oil	
½ a white onion, thinly sliced	*2* Heat the coconut oil over medium heat in a sauté pan. Sauté the onions until translucent. Add the garlic, lemongrass puree, and ginger and sauté for 1 to 2 minutes until fragrant.
2 cloves garlic, crushed	
1-inch piece of fresh ginger, grated (about 1 tablespoon)	
1 pound boneless, skinless chicken thighs, cut into 1-inch chunks	*3* Sprinkle the chicken with the salt and pepper and add it to the pan. Brown the chicken on all sides, adding more coconut oil if needed.
1 teaspoon sea salt	
½ teaspoon pepper	*4* Stir in the green curry paste, coating all the chicken. Add the rest of the vegetables and the kaffir lime leaves and cook for 2 minutes.
2 tablespoons green curry paste	
1 small zucchini, sliced	
1 red bell pepper, sliced	*5* Add the coconut milk and simmer on low for 15 minutes or until the chicken is cooked through and the vegetables are cooked but still firm and colorful.
2 cups white mushrooms, sliced	
4 kaffir lime leaves, chopped	
2 cups coconut milk	*6* Top with the basil and serve.
½ cup fresh basil, chopped	

Per serving: Calories 473 (From Fat 335); Fat 37g (Saturated 28g); Cholesterol 95mg; Sodium 737mg; Carbohydrate 13g (Dietary Fiber 2.5g); Protein 27g.

*N*ote: Kaffir lime leaf, also known as lime leaf, is a key ingredient in Thai cooking as well as other Southeast-Asian cuisines. Your local grocery store may carry Thai Kitchen brand lime leaves and green curry paste, or you can look for these items at an Asian market.

Recipe courtesy Arsy Vartanian, author of Rubies & Radishes (www.rubiesandradishes.com)

This recipe has been vetted by the team at Whole9 (http://whole9life.com) and is considered acceptable for a cleansing 30-day Paleo launch.

Sun-Dried Tomato and Basil Stuffed Chicken Breast

Prep time: 20 min • **Cook time:** 30 min • **Yield:** 2 servings

Ingredients	Directions
2 boneless, skinless chicken breasts **Salt and pepper** **2 cloves garlic, crushed** **2 teaspoons pine nuts** **4 sun-dried tomatoes, marinated in olive oil, chopped (about 2 tablespoons)** **¼ cup fresh basil, chopped** **1 to 2 tablespoons ghee** **½ cup chicken stock**	*1* Place the chicken breasts between two pieces of waxed paper and beat with a meat mallet or rolling pin until they're thin enough to roll. Slice thick chicken breasts horizontally almost all the way through and open them flat before pounding. *2* Salt and pepper both sides of the chicken breasts. In the center of each breast, place 1 clove of garlic, 1 teaspoon of the pine nuts, half the sun-dried tomatoes, and half the basil. *3* Starting at the broader end, roll the chicken around the filling and secure with a toothpick.

4   Heat the ghee in a skillet with a tight-fitting lid. Brown the stuffed chicken breasts on all sides.

5   Add the chicken stock to the skillet, cover, and lower the heat. Simmer for 20 to 25 minutes or until the chicken is cooked through.

6   Remove the chicken from skillet and cover with foil to keep warm.

7   Turn up the heat under the skillet until the sauce is boiling and then reduce heat to low and allow the sauce to reduce uncovered to your desired consistency. Pour the sauce over the chicken and serve.

Per serving: *Calories 216 (From Fat 74); Fat 8g (Saturated 2g); Cholesterol 81mg; Sodium 415mg; Carbohydrate 4g (Dietary Fiber 0.5g); Protein 30g.*

Note: Organic chicken breasts are smaller and thinner and therefore won't require pounding in Step 1.

Note: You can find a ghee recipe in Chapter 9.

Recipe courtesy Arsy Vartanian, author of Rubies & Radishes (www.rubiesandradishes.com)

This recipe has been vetted by the team at Whole9 (http://whole9life.com) and is considered acceptable for a cleansing 30-day Paleo launch.

Chili Lime Barbecued Chicken

Prep time: 10 min, plus marinating time • **Cook time:** 30 min • **Yield:** 6 servings

Ingredients	Directions
1 medium chicken (about 3.5 lbs)	*1* Split the chicken in half and press it down to flatten it.
1 tablespoon chili powder	*2* In a large container, combine the chicken, chili powder, lime zest, cilantro, garlic, and olive oil. Season lightly with salt and pepper and mix well, using your hands, until the chicken is uniformly covered in marinade.
3 limes, zested and halved	
¼ cup chopped fresh cilantro	
4 cloves garlic, minced	*3* Marinate in the refrigerator for 30 minutes to 24 hours.
1 tablespoon olive oil	
Kosher salt	*4* When you're ready to cook the chicken, preheat your grill to 300 degrees, using lump charcoal if possible.
Pepper	
	5 Lay the chicken skin side up on a sheet pan and season with salt and pepper. Transfer the chicken to the grill, skin side down, and squeeze one lime half over both pieces of chicken.

6 Cook the chicken with the grill lid closed for about 20 minutes, basting with lime juice twice during cooking, until the bottom is nicely browned. (Use one lime half per basting.)

7 Sprinkle the top side with salt and flip the chicken over. Squeeze with lime juice as in Step 5 and repeat Step 6, cooking until the thickest part of the breast reaches an internal temperature of 165 degrees (about 15 minutes).

8 Remove the chicken from the grill and let it rest for a few minutes before serving.

Per serving: *Calories 593 (From Fat 378); Fat 42g (Saturated 12g); Cholesterol 198mg; Sodium 188mg; Carbohydrate 4g (Dietary Fiber 1g); Protein 49g.*

Note: This recipe is a great make-ahead protein option. You can store it in the fridge for up to a week or in the freezer for up to six months. If you're going to freeze it, do so immediately.

Tip: To help flatten the chicken on the grill, use a weight (such as a brick covered in foil and lightly greased). The weight helps get a good sear on the skin side, but you do have to remove it to baste with limes.

*Recipe courtesy Nick Massie, chef and author of Paleo Nick (*http://paleonick.com*)*

*This recipe has been vetted by the team at Whole9 (*http://whole9life.com*) and is considered acceptable for a cleansing 30-day Paleo launch.*

Tandoori Chicken Thighs

Prep time: 10 min, plus marinating time • **Cook time:** 40 min • **Yield:** 6 servings

Ingredients	Directions

Ingredients

4 pounds bone-in, skin-on chicken thighs

Kosher salt

Pepper

1 cup coconut milk

1½ tablespoons tandoori seasoning

4 limes

1 tablespoon coconut oil

Directions

1 Liberally season the chicken with salt and pepper in a large bowl.

2 Combine the coconut milk, tandoori seasoning, and the juice of 1 lime in a large zip-top bag; mix well. Add the chicken to the bag, shake it around to coat, and marinate in the fridge for 8 hours.

3 When you're ready to cook the chicken, preheat the oven to 400 degrees. Place a wire rack on a foil-lined rimmed baking tray and grease the rack with coconut oil.

4 Arrange the chicken skin-side down on the rack and bake for 20 minutes. Flip the pieces over and bake for another 20 minutes until it has some charred bits.

5 Cut the remaining limes into wedges. The chicken is done when the juices run clear when you pierce the meat with a fork or knife near the bone. Serve immediately with the lime wedges.

Per serving: Calories 774 (From Fat 525); Fat 58g (Saturated 22g); Cholesterol 227mg; Sodium 301mg; Carbohydrate 6g (Dietary Fiber 1.5g); Protein 57g.

Tip: You can throw this simple Indian dish together in 10 minutes and leave it to marinate while you're at work; the chicken will be ready to bake when you get home.

*Recipe courtesy Michelle Tam, author of Nom Nom Paleo (*http://nomnompaleo.com*)*

*This recipe has been vetted by the team at Whole9 (*http://whole9life.com*) and is considered acceptable for a cleansing 30-day Paleo launch.*

Slow-Roasted Rack of Lamb

Prep time: 10 min, plus resting time • **Cook time:** 60–90 min • **Yield:** 2 servings

Ingredients	Directions
2-pound rack of lamb **Kosher salt** **3 tablespoons dukkah** **Pepper**	*1* Dry the lamb thoroughly with paper towels. Liberally sprinkle it all over with salt and refrigerate it for 4 hours to 2 days.
	2 Remove the lamb from the fridge at least 1 hour before you cook it. Preheat the oven to 250 degrees, with the oven rack set in the middle. Place a wire rack on a foil-lined baking tray.
	3 Coat the lamb with the dukkah and the pepper and place it on the wire rack.
	4 Insert an instant-read, in-oven thermometer probe into the thickest part of the lamb. Aim it toward the center, away from the rib bones. Place the lamb in the oven.
	5 Bake for 60 to 90 minutes. Remove the lamb as soon as the thermometer registers 130 degrees for medium rare or 140 degrees for medium.
	6 Remove the lamb from the oven and let rest for 15 minutes. Slice between the ribs before serving.

Per serving: Calories 928 (From Fat 374); Fat 42g (Saturated 15g); Cholesterol 417mg; Sodium 568mg; Carbohydrate 0.5g (Dietary Fiber 0.5g); Protein 129g.

Note: Dukkah is an Egyptian spice blend. Chapter 15 has a recipe for homemade dukkah.

Tip: Instant-read, in-oven thermometers let you keep track of your food temperature without having to continually open and close the oven (letting out heat). I talk more about meat thermometers in Chapter 21.

Recipe courtesy Michelle Tam, author of Nom Nom Paleo (http://nomnompaleo.com)

This recipe has been vetted by the team at Whole9 (http://whole9life.com) and is considered acceptable for a cleansing 30-day Paleo launch.

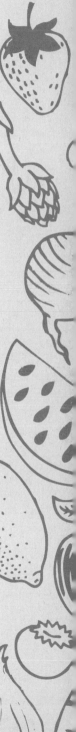

Chocolate Chili

Prep time: 20 min • **Cook time:** 2–3 hr • **Yield:** 8 servings

Ingredients	Directions
2 tablespoons coconut oil	**1** Heat a large, deep pot over medium-high heat and add the coconut oil. When the oil is melted, add the onions and, stirring with a wooden spoon, cook until they're translucent, about 7 minutes.
2 medium onions, diced (about 2 cups)	
4 cloves garlic, minced (about 4 teaspoons)	**2** Add the garlic and, as soon as it's fragrant (about 30 seconds), crumble the ground beef into the pan with your hands, mixing with the wooden spoon to combine. Continue to cook the meat, stirring often, until it's no longer pink.
2 pounds ground beef	
1 teaspoon dried oregano	
2 tablespoons chili powder	
2 tablespoons ground cumin	**3** In a small bowl, crush the oregano between your palms to release its flavor. Add the chili powder, cumin, cocoa powder, allspice, and salt. Mix with a fork and then stir into the ground beef.
1½ tablespoons unsweetened cocoa powder	
1 teaspoon ground allspice	
1 teaspoon Celtic sea salt	**4** Add the tomato paste and stir until combined, about 2 minutes.
One 6-ounce can tomato paste	
One 14.5-ounce can fire-roasted chopped tomatoes	**5** Add the tomatoes with their juice, the beef broth, and 1 cup of water to the pot. Stir well. Bring to a boil and then reduce the heat and simmer uncovered for at least 2 hours.
One 14.5-ounce can beef broth	

Per serving: Calories 472 (From Fat 342); Fat 38g (Saturated 16g); Cholesterol 88mg; Sodium 1,056mg; Carbohydrate 14g (Dietary Fiber 3g); Protein 20g.

Recipe courtesy Melissa Joulwan, author of Well Fed: Paleo Recipes for People Who Love to Eat and The Clothes Make the Girl (www.theclothesmakethegirl.com)

This recipe has been vetted by the team at Whole9 (http://whole9life.com) and is considered acceptable for a cleansing 30-day Paleo launch.

Spicy Stuffed Eggplant

Prep time: 10 min • **Cook time:** 20 min • **Yield:** 4 servings

Ingredients	*Directions*
2 large eggplants	*1* Preheat the oven to 400 degrees.
5 tablespoons olive oil, divided	*2* Wash the eggplants and cut them in half lengthwise. Remove the pulp, chop it coarsely, and set it aside. Leave a scooped shell about ½-inch thick.
1 onion chopped	
2 cloves garlic, minced	
One 14.5-ounce can diced tomatoes, drained	*3* In a large skillet, heat half the oil. Place the eggplant shells cut-side down in the oil and cook for about 5 minutes. With tongs, transfer the shells cut side up to a shallow, ovenproof dish.
One 8-ounce can tomato sauce	
½ teaspoon dried thyme	*4* Add the remaining oil to the skillet and sauté the onions and garlic for 2 minutes over medium heat.
½ teaspoon ground cayenne pepper	
Pinch of salt	*5* Add the eggplant pulp, tomatoes, tomato sauce, thyme, cayenne, salt, and pepper and cook over medium heat until most of the moisture evaporates and a stew-like mixture remains.
Pinch of pepper	
½ pound ground beef, cooked	
2 tablespoons chopped fresh parsley	*6* Remove the skillet from the heat and mix in the beef. Stuff the eggplant shells with the meat mixture and bake for 15 minutes.
	7 Top with the parsley and serve.

Per serving: Calories 539 (From Fat 356); Fat 40g (Saturated 7g); Cholesterol 38mg; Sodium 306mg; Carbohydrate 33g (Dietary Fiber 10g); Protein 21g.

Recipe courtesy Mark Sisson, author of Primal Blueprint and Mark's Daily Apple (www. marksdailyapple.com)

This recipe has been vetted by the team at Whole9 (http://whole9life.com) and is considered acceptable for a cleansing 30-day Paleo launch.

Beef Stuffed Zucchini

Prep time: 25 min • **Cook time:** 30 min • **Yield:** 8 servings

Ingredients	Directions
4 large zucchini	*1* Preheat the oven to 350 degrees.
2 pounds ground beef	
3 cloves garlic, crushed	*2* Cut the zucchini in half lengthwise and scoop out the seeds. Chop about half the seeds for the stuffing and put them in a large bowl; discard the remainder. Place the zucchini shells in a shallow baking dish.
1 tablespoon coconut aminos	
1 large shallot, minced	
¼ cup fresh flat-leaf parsley, chopped	*3* Add the ground beef, garlic, coconut aminos, shallot, parsley, chili powder, egg, salt, and pepper to the zucchini pulp and mix well.
1 teaspoon chipotle chili powder	
1 egg, beaten	*4* Sauté the meat mixture in a large sauté pan until the meat is lightly browned.
1½ teaspoons sea salt	
1 teaspoon pepper	*5* Divide the meat mixture among the zucchini halves, piling the filling up over the top of each shell.
	6 Bake for approximately 30 minutes or until the zucchini flesh is tender. The zucchini gets very soft after baking, so be extra careful when serving.

Per serving: Calories 330 (From Fat 168); Fat 19g (Saturated 7g); Cholesterol 98mg; Sodium 386mg; Carbohydrate 10g (Dietary Fiber 3g); Protein 31g.

Vary It! You can easily substitute bell peppers for the zucchini in this recipe.

Tip: Garnish the zucchini boats with the Fried Sage Leaves from Chapter 10 before serving.

Recipe courtesy Arsy Vartanian, author of Rubies & Radishes (www.rubiesandradishes.com)

This recipe has been vetted by the team at Whole9 (http://whole9life.com) and is considered acceptable for a cleansing 30-day Paleo launch.

Chapter 15

Paleo Perfect Spice Blends

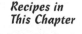
In This Chapter

▶ Utilizing spices that heal the body

▶ Stirring up spice blends to make your meals pop

Think about all the little things that make a big impact in your life — a simple walk on the beach or maybe a smile from someone you love. Well, spices are kind of like that: just small things that make a big difference.

Spices crank up the flavor in any dish. Bursting with sweetness or warming with heat, spices turn the ordinary into the extraordinary. Adding spices lets you create really great dishes with few ingredients; the spices take away the need to add a lot of extras like rich sauces and condiments.

Cayenne pepper, chili pepper, chipotle powder, and paprika are considered *nightshades.* This label means that if you have an autoimmune or inflammatory condition, these spices may aggravate your symptoms, and you should avoid them.

Tapping the Healing Power of Spices

Many cultures have used spices to heal for thousands of years. That's why I love to add lots of spices to my meals; in fact, my spice drawer is probably the busiest drawer in my kitchen! The following are my top picks for healing spices:

✔ **Cinnamon:** Cinnamon is serious about balancing blood sugar. Its active ingredient, *cinnamaldehyde,* decreases blood sugar, total cholesterol, and triglycerides and increases good cholesterol. This wonderful spice may also help treat cancer because it may slow the development of new blood supplies to tumors.

- **Cayenne:** Cayenne lowers blood pressure and has even been known to stop a heart attack! Cayenne thins phlegm and eases its passage through the lungs, and it improves digestion and relieves nausea and gas.

- **Black pepper:** Pepper is a great spice to maximize your digestion. It helps move food along the colon at a good pace, and the quicker and smoother the ride, the healthier your colon.

  If you have digestive complaints, black pepper can be irritating to the intestinal lining.

- **Turmeric:** The active ingredient in turmeric is *curcumin,* which has been shown to protect and heal virtually every organ in the human body. Turmeric protects against cancer, Alzheimer's disease, Parkinson's disease, heart disease, stroke, diabetes, eye diseases, depression, and skin problems. Research at Tufts University showed that turmeric may prevent weight gain.

- **Curry:** If you've ever tasted Indian food, you've probably tried curry. It controls diabetes and can prevent or treat heart disease, infection, age-related memory loss, and inflammation. Curry has powerful antioxidants called *carbazole alkaloids* that are abundant only in the curry leaf and are responsible for preventing cell damage, which causes disease and premature aging.

- **Oregano:** Oregano is your natural protection against infection. The active compounds in oregano have strong antiviral, antibacterial, and antifungal properties. Oregano helps get rid of intestinal parasites and kills the bacteria that causes food poisoning; it heals ulcers, calms intestinal irritation, and aids in digestion. Plus, oregano contains a lot of minerals, antioxidants, fiber, and omega-3 fatty acids.

- **Parsley:** Parsley contains an antioxidant called *apigenin* that helps other antioxidants work better. Parsley is used as a diuretic; can reduce high blood pressure; and is a natural agent to fight cancer, heart disease, and Type 2 diabetes.

- **Thyme:** The healing oil in thyme is a natural antiseptic. When applied to skin or the mucous membranes of the mouth, it kills germs. Thyme is great for calming coughs and helping prevent tooth decay and general infection.

- **Ginger:** Ginger rules all natural digestive aids: It relieves nausea and vomiting, settles the stomach, and eases the discomfort from gas and bloating. Research shows that ginger is one of the most effective remedies available for motion sickness, even more so than over-the-counter medications. It's also an antioxidant, antibacterial, antiviral, and anti-inflammatory and helps treat migraine headaches, arthritis, and asthma.

Succulent Steak Seasoning

Prep time: 5 min • **Yield:** ½ cup

Ingredients	Directions
2 tablespoons pepper	**1** Combine all ingredients in a container or jar (preferably glass) with a tight-fitting lid. Store in a cool, dark place, shaking the jar well to distribute the spices between uses.
2 tablespoons salt	
1 tablespoon powered garlic	
½ teaspoon curry powder	
½ teaspoon apple cider vinegar	**2** Rub the seasoning well into meat before baking, grilling, or slow cooking.
4 tablespoons dry mustard	
1 teaspoon Celtic sea salt	

Per serving: Calories 23 (From Fat 11); Fat 1g (Saturated 0g); Cholesterol 0mg; Sodium 1,904mg; Carbohydrate 2.5g (Dietary Fiber 1g); Protein 1g.

Note: This spice blend really pops with grass-fed meats because they're incredibly lean.

This recipe has been vetted by the team at Whole9 (`http://whole9life.com`) and is considered acceptable for a cleansing 30-day Paleo launch.

Everything Seafood Seasoning

Prep time: 5 min • **Yield:** 1½ tablespoons

Ingredients	*Directions*
2 teaspoons celery salt	*1* Combine all ingredients in a container or jar (preferably glass) with a tight-fitting lid. Store in a cool, dark place, shaking the jar well to distribute the spices between uses.
½ teaspoon paprika	
¼ teaspoon pepper	
¼ teaspoon cayenne pepper	
¼ teaspoon dry mustard	*2* Rub the seasoning well into fish or seafood before baking, grilling, or slow cooking.
¼ teaspoon ground nutmeg	
¼ teaspoon ground cinnamon	
¼ teaspoon ground cardamom	
¼ teaspoon ground allspice	
¼ teaspoon ground ginger	

Per serving: Calories 3 (From Fat 0); Fat 0g (Saturated 0g); Cholesterol 0mg; Sodium 0.5mg; Carbohydrate 0.5g (Dietary Fiber 0.5g); Protein 0g.

Note: This spice blend is a home run on seafood, but it works on many other dishes as well, so feel free to experiment.

This recipe has been vetted by the team at Whole9 (http://whole9life.com) and is considered acceptable for a cleansing 30-day Paleo launch.

Dukkah

Prep time: 5 min • **Cook time:** 10 min • **Yield:** 1 cup

Ingredients	Directions
⅓ **cup raw hazelnuts**	**1** Preheat the oven to 375 degrees.
¼ **cup roasted shelled pistachios**	**2** Spread the hazelnuts on a foil-lined baking sheet and roast them for 5 to 7 minutes or until they turn golden brown and fragrant.
⅓ **cup raw sesame seeds**	
¼ **cup coriander seeds**	**3** Transfer the roasted hazelnuts to a clean towel and allow them to cool. Use the towel to rub off the papery hazelnut skins and discard them. Transfer the skinned hazelnuts to a medium bowl and add the pistachios.
2 tablespoons cumin seeds	
	4 Toast the sesame seeds in a dry skillet over medium-low heat for 1 minute or until they turn light brown, shaking constantly to prevent scorching. Reserve 1 tablespoon of the toasted seeds; place the rest in the bowl with the nuts.
	5 Toast the coriander seeds in the skillet until they're fragrant and place them in the bowl. Repeat with the cumin seeds.
	6 When the mixture of nuts and seeds has cooled, coarsely grind it in small batches in a spice grinder until lightly crushed. Mix in the reserved toasted sesame seeds. Store the spice blend in an airtight container in the fridge for up to 3 months.

Per serving: Calories 72 (From Fat 57); Fat 6g (Saturated 0.5g); Cholesterol 0mg; Sodium 3mg; Carbohydrate 3.5g (Dietary Fiber 2g); Protein 2g.

Note: Dukkah is an Egyptian spice blend that adds a smoky, nutty flavor to roasts in particular.

*Recipe courtesy Michelle Tam, author of Nom Nom Paleo (*http://nomnompaleo.com*)*

*This recipe has been vetted by the team at Whole9 (*http://whole9life.com*) and is considered acceptable for a cleansing 30-day Paleo launch.*

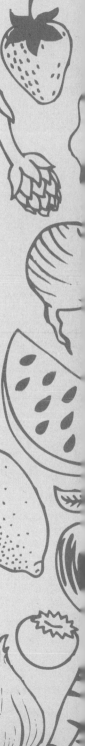

Flame Out Blend

Prep time: 5 min • **Yield:** ⅓ cup

Ingredients	*Directions*
2 tablespoons ground cinnamon	**1** Combine all ingredients in a container or jar (preferably glass) with a tight-fitting lid.
2 tablespoons ground ginger	
1 tablespoon orange zest	**2** Store in the refrigerator for up to 3 months.
1 tablespoon lemon zest	

Per serving: Calories 10 (From Fat 0); Fat 0g (Saturated 0g); Cholesterol 0mg; Sodium 0.5mg; Carbohydrate 2.5g (Dietary Fiber 1.5g); Protein 0g.

Note: This spice blend is fantastic if you suffer from any kind of inflammatory or autoimmune conditions. The ginger helps your body cool down. You can use this spice anywhere you want a cooling blend, but it's particularly good in baking!

This recipe has been vetted by the team at Whole9 (http://whole9life.com) and is considered acceptable for a cleansing 30-day Paleo launch.

Italian Seasoning

Prep time: 5 min • **Yield:** ¾ cup

Ingredients	*Directions*
3 tablespoons dried basil	**1** Combine all ingredients in a container or jar (preferably glass) with a tight-fitting lid. Store in a cool, dark place for up to 6 months, shaking the jar well to distribute the spices between uses.
3 tablespoons dried oregano	
3 tablespoons dried parsley	
2 tablespoons dried marjoram	
1 tablespoon garlic powder	
1 teaspoon onion powder	
1 teaspoon dried thyme	
1 teaspoon dried rosemary	
¼ teaspoon pepper	
¼ teaspoon red pepper flakes	

Per serving: Calories 7 (From Fat 0); Fat 0g (Saturated 0g); Cholesterol 0mg; Sodium 1.5mg; Carbohydrate 1.5g (Dietary Fiber 1g); Protein 0.5g.

This recipe has been vetted by the team at Whole9 (http://whole9life.com) and is considered acceptable for a cleansing 30-day Paleo launch.

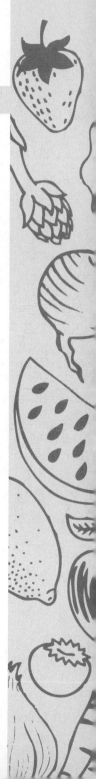

Gremolata

Prep time: 15 min • **Cook time:** 5 min • **Yield:** ⅔ cup

Ingredients

1 bunch Italian parsley, stems removed

Zest of 3 lemons

4 cloves garlic, minced (about 2 teaspoons)

½ cup olive oil

Kosher salt to taste

Pepper to taste

1 tablespoon lemon juice

Directions

1 Combine the parsley, lemon zest, and garlic in a blender. With the blender running, slowly drizzle in the olive oil. Blend until the consistency is slightly thicker than pickle relish, adding more parsley or using less olive oil as necessary.

2 Season with the salt, pepper, and lemon juice and enjoy!

Per serving: Calories 82 (From Fat 81); Fat 9g (Saturated 1.5g); Cholesterol 0mg; Sodium 42mg; Carbohydrate 0.5g (Dietary Fiber 0g); Protein 0g.

Note: *Gremolata* is a basic spice blend that's a great compliment to many entrees and is particularly lovely with seafood dishes.

Tip: Instead of a blender, you can also bash the ingredients in a mortar and pestle, drizzling in the olive oil as you do.

Recipe courtesy Nick Massie, chef and author of Paleo Nick (`http://paleonick.com`)

This recipe has been vetted by the team at Whole9 (`http://whole9life.com`) and is considered acceptable for a cleansing 30-day Paleo launch.

Chapter 16

Namaste! Paleo Vegetarian Sides

I f you're one of those people who just can't seem to get onboard with eating your vegetables, I'll give you one solid reason why you should embrace vegetables as if they were the shiniest gift under the tree: Eating vegetables boosts your immunity. Everything rises and falls on your immune system. When it's strong, you avoid the pitfalls of disease, and your body expresses vitality and health.

Vegetables provide *super immunity,* which occurs when your body's greatest protector (your immune system) is working to the best of its ability to get and keep you well. Super immunity can even save your life, protecting you from the simplest of challenges, such as the common cold, to the most threatening, such as cancer.

Paleo vegetables differ from other vegetables because they work best with your body to create health and provide the most nutrients. Contrast that with non-Paleo vegetables such as corn (which is also a grain) and white potatoes (which cause an unfavorable insulin reaction).

No matter what your health goals are — getting well, staying well, losing weight, or fighting aging — attaining them starts with creating the healthiest cells possible. Discovering foods like the vegetarian side dishes in this chapter helps your body produce these healthy cells. You can find bonus recipes, including one for a comforting Zucchini and Tomato Bake, online at www. dummies.com/extras/paleocookbook.

Striving for nutrient density

Nutritional excellence happens when you eat foods with *high nutrient density,* which means they have a lot of nutrients in relation to the amount of calories they contain. Unfortunately, the average American takes in about 60 percent of his calories from *low nutrient density foods* — processed foods that have added flavors, colors, sweeteners, and rancid oils and are a gluten-filled, flour-loaded dietary mess. When you eat these foods, you weaken your healing shield and open yourself up to disease and premature aging.

High nutrient density foods are the mainstay of the Paleo lifestyle. All the recipes in this chapter (and in this book, for that matter) provide you with the highest nutrient density foods on the planet.

When you think of vegetables, think of the rainbow. You want to get as many colors in your diet as you can. The brighter the color, the more nutrients the veggies contain.

Understanding How Vegetables Keep You Looking Young

Healthy cells are different from cells under *oxidative stress,* which have unstable molecules, damage tissue, and age you. To avoid premature aging and turn back the hands of time, you have to eliminate the oxidative stress patterns placed on your body. You can do so by eating immune-boosting, nutrient-dense foods such as Paleo vegetables. (Check out the nearby sidebar "Striving for nutrient density" for details on this designation.)

When you begin eating foods with nutritional excellence, your body starts to shed all its unhealthy cells. Layers of fat begin to peel away; you become leaner, stronger, and disease-free and defy your age. Immune-boosting foods do all these things and more:

- ✔ Contain lots of minerals, helping your cells work their best
- ✔ Contain the vitamins your body needs in sufficient amounts so you aren't in a deficient state, which leaves you wide open for disease
- ✔ Add robust amounts of fiber to your daily plate for intestinal health

If vegetables have been missing from your plate lately, start by adding just one vegetable to every meal. As you figure out what Paleo vegetables you like and what recipes you love, work up to two vegetables on every plate.

Cocoa Cauliflower

Prep time: 5 min • **Cook time:** 40 min • **Yield:** 4 servings

Ingredients	Directions
1 head fresh cauliflower	**1** Preheat the oven to 400 degrees. Cover a baking sheet with parchment paper or aluminum foil.
1 teaspoon paprika	
1 teaspoon unsweetened cocoa powder	**2** With a sharp knife, remove the core of the cauliflower and break the head into florets. Place the florets in a large mixing bowl.
¼ teaspoon salt	
¼ teaspoon pepper	**3** In a small, microwave-safe bowl, mix the paprika, cocoa, salt, pepper, and garlic with a fork. Add the coconut oil and microwave for 15 to 20 seconds, until the coconut oil is melted and the spices are fragrant.
1 clove garlic, minced	
2 tablespoons coconut oil	
	4 Drizzle the spiced oil over the cauliflower in the bowl and toss until well coated.
	5 Spread the cauliflower in a single layer on the baking sheet and roast in the oven for about 25 to 30 minutes, until it's tender and beginning to brown.

Per serving: Calories 81 (From Fat 63); Fat 7g (Saturated 6g); Cholesterol 0mg; Sodium 168mg; Carbohydrate 5g (Dietary Fiber 2g); Protein 2g.

Tip: If you don't care for the somewhat-bitter taste of unsweetened cocoa, you can make this dish without it; the cauliflower will still be tasty!

*Recipe courtesy Melissa Joulwan, author of Well Fed: Paleo Recipes for People Who Love to Eat and The Clothes Make the Girl (*www.theclothesmakethegirl.com*)*

*This recipe has been vetted by the team at Whole9 (*http://whole9life.com*) and is considered acceptable for a cleansing 30-day Paleo launch.*

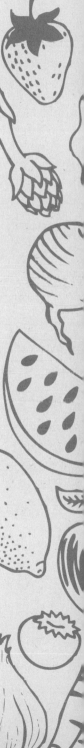

Italian Broccoli

Prep time: 5 min • **Cook time:** 20 min • **Yield:** 4 servings

Ingredients	Directions
¼ cup macadamia nut oil or coconut oil	**1** Heat the oil in a large skillet over medium heat.
2 cloves garlic, crushed	**2** Add the garlic and cook for a few minutes, stirring constantly.
One 14.5-ounce can diced tomatoes	
1 tablespoon balsamic vinegar	**3** Pour in the tomatoes with their juices, the vinegar, and the basil and simmer until the liquid has reduced by about half.
¼ teaspoon dried basil	
1 pound broccoli, trimmed and cut into spears	**4** Place the broccoli on top of the tomatoes and season with a little salt and pepper.
Salt and pepper to taste	
	5 Cover and simmer over low heat for 10 minutes or until the broccoli is tender. Don't overcook the broccoli; it should be a vibrant green.
	6 Pour the cooked broccoli into a serving dish and toss to blend with the sauce before serving.

Per serving: _Calories 180 (From Fat 126); Fat 14g (Saturated 12g); Cholesterol 0mg; Sodium 196mg; Carbohydrate 14g (Dietary Fiber 4g); Protein 4g._

Tip: If you use coconut oil, the dish will take on a bit of coconut flavor. If you use the macadamia nut oil, it will have a richer, buttery taste.

This recipe has been vetted by the team at Whole9 (http://whole9life.com) _and is considered acceptable for a cleansing 30-day Paleo launch._

Creamy Kale

Prep time: 5 min • **Cook time:** 10 min • **Yield:** 2 servings

Ingredients	Directions
1 large bunch kale (about 12 leaves)	**1** Wash the kale and shake off any excess water. Remove the tough stems with the tip of a sharp knife. Roughly chop or tear the leaves.
1 teaspoon ground cumin	
½ teaspoon ground coriander	**2** Heat a large skillet over medium-high heat. Toss in about half the kale. Stir with a wooden spoon until the kale begins to wilt, and then add the remaining kale. Stir and cover with a lid.
2 cloves garlic, crushed	
Pinch of salt	
1 teaspoon coconut oil	**3** In a small bowl, mix the cumin, coriander, garlic, and salt. Set aside.
½ cup coconut milk	
	4 When the kale is dark green and beginning to wilt, remove the lid and let any remaining water evaporate.
	5 When the pan is mostly dry, push the kale to the side and add the coconut oil. Let the oil heat and then pour the spices directly into the pool of oil to release their fragrance, about 20 seconds.
	6 Pour the coconut milk into the pan (not directly into the oil), stirring to combine the kale, seasonings, and milk. Sauté until the sauce begins to thicken.

Per serving: *Calories 131 (From Fat 90); Fat 10g (Saturated 8g); Cholesterol 0mg; Sodium 58mg; Carbohydrate 10g (Dietary Fiber 2g); Protein 3g.*

Tip: You can substitute another sturdy leafy green for the kale.

*Recipe courtesy Melissa Joulwan, author of Well Fed: Paleo Recipes for People Who Love to Eat and The Clothes Make the Girl (*www.theclothesmakethegirl.com*)*

*This recipe has been vetted by the team at Whole9 (*http://whole9life.com*) and is considered acceptable for a cleansing 30-day Paleo launch.*

Baked Sweet Potatoes

Prep time: 10 min • **Cook time:** 30 min • **Yield:** 4 servings

Ingredients	Directions
3 sweet potatoes, peeled and cubed (about 2 cups)	*1* Cover the sweet potatoes with water in a large stockpot. Bring to a boil and cook until the potatoes are fork tender, about 15 minutes. Drain and transfer to a large mixing bowl or stand mixer.
1.2 ounces freeze-dried blueberries, or ½ cup fresh blueberries	
¼ cup coconut milk	*2* Preheat the oven to 400 degrees.
2 tablespoons lemon juice	*3* If you're using freeze-dried blueberries, pulse them in a food processor to make a powder and then add it to your sweet potatoes. If you're using fresh blueberries, don't add them yet.
2 tablespoons unsalted butter	
1 tablespoon honey	
1 teaspoon ground cinnamon	
¼ cup chopped pecans	*4* Add the coconut milk, lemon juice, butter, honey, and cinnamon to the potatoes and use the stand mixer or a hand mixer to beat the potatoes until no lumps remain.
	5 If you're using fresh blueberries, fold them into the mashed potatoes by hand.
	6 Transfer the potato mixture to four small ramekins and sprinkle the pecans on top. Place the ramekins on a cookie sheet and bake for 10 to 15 minutes or until the pecans are toasted but not burned.
	7 Serve alone or with a scoop of refrigerated or frozen coconut milk.

Per serving: Calories 228 (From Fat 117); Fat 13g (Saturated 6g); Cholesterol 15mg; Sodium 62mg; Carbohydrate 29g (Dietary Fiber 4g); Protein 3g.

Vary It! If you can find purple sweet potatoes, substitute them for the regular sweet potatoes for a nice change.

*Recipe courtesy George Bryant, CEO and author of Civilized Caveman Cooking Creations (*http://civilizedcavemancooking.com*)*

Sautéed Kohlrabi

Prep time: 10 min • **Cook time:** 10 min • **Yield:** 2 servings

Ingredients	*Directions*
2 kohlrabies	*1* Trim the stalks from the kohlrabies and slice off the bottoms. Peel the bulbs and cut into ¼-inch-thick slices.
1 tablespoon butter	
2 cloves garlic, crushed	
Pinch of salt	*2* Bring a pot of water to a boil. Add the kohlrabies and cook until tender but still firm, about 4 to 5 minutes. Drain the kohlrabies and run them under cold water to stop the cooking. Dry them on a paper towel.
Pinch of pepper	
Chopped parsley for garnish	
	3 Heat the butter in a large skillet and add the garlic. Sauté until fragrant, stirring constantly. Add the kohlrabies to the skillet, along with the salt and pepper, and sauté until they're golden brown on both sides.
	4 Sprinkle with the parsley and serve.

Per serving: Calories 92 (From Fat 54); Fat 6g (Saturated 4g); Cholesterol 15mg; Sodium 319mg; Carbohydrate 10g (Dietary Fiber 5g); Protein 3g.

*Recipe courtesy Arsy Vartanian, author of Rubies & Radishes (*www.rubiesandradishes.com*)*

*This recipe has been vetted by the team at Whole9 (*http://whole9life.com*) and is considered acceptable for a cleansing 30-day Paleo launch.*

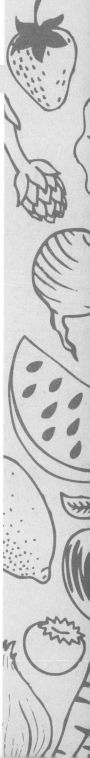

Brussels Sprouts with Cranberries and Almonds

Prep time: 10 min • **Cook time:** 30 min • **Yield:** 4 servings

Ingredients	Directions
3 tablespoons coconut oil	**1** Preheat a large skillet on medium-low heat for 1 to 2 minutes. Add the coconut oil.
1 medium onion, chopped	
2 cloves garlic, minced	**2** Add the onions and garlic and season with the salt and pepper. Cook for a few minutes until the onions are translucent.
Pinch of salt, plus more to taste	
Pinch of pepper, plus more to taste	**3** Add the Brussels sprouts and stir to thoroughly coat with the oil. Sauté, adding more oil if the pan starts to dry out and brown. After a couple of minutes, add the almonds, cranberries, and flaxseed (if desired).
4 cups Brussels sprouts, trimmed and sliced	
½ cup almonds, chopped	
¼ cup dried cranberries (no sugar added)	**4** Stir thoroughly and cook until the sprouts are lightly caramelized. Salt and pepper to taste.
Pinch of flaxseed (optional)	

Per serving: Calories 265 (From Fat 180); Fat 20g (Saturated 10g); Cholesterol 0mg; Sodium 129mg; Carbohydrate 21g (Dietary Fiber 6g); Protein 7g.

Vary It! Try adding chopped celery and napa cabbage to the sprouts for a different flavor and texture.

Tip: You can use this fabulous vegetable dish as the foundation for many different meals, so make extra! Not only is it a great side dish, but it's also an awesome meal. Add grilled chicken or steak or top with eggs.

*This recipe has been vetted by the team at Whole9 (*http://whole9life.com*) and is considered acceptable for a cleansing 30-day Paleo launch.*

Kimchi

Prep time: 10 min, plus marinating time • **Yield:** 6 servings

Ingredients	Directions
1 medium to large napa cabbage, shredded	**1** Toss all the ingredients together in a mixing bowl. Cover and allow the mixture to sit in a cool, dark place overnight or for at least a few hours for the flavors to mingle.
1 cup shredded carrot	
½ cup diced red bell peppers	
½ cup shredded onion	**2** After the mixture is done marinating, serve immediately. Store any leftovers in the fridge for 5 to 7 days.
1 tablespoon apple cider vinegar	
1 tablespoon minced ginger	
1 teaspoon honey	
¼ teaspoon red chile flakes	
1 tablespoon salt	

Per serving: Calories 26 (From Fat 0); Fat 0g (Saturated 0g); Cholesterol 0mg; Sodium 1,180mg; Carbohydrate 6g (Dietary Fiber 1g); Protein 1g.

Note: Kimchi is an Asian pickled condiment. It really works at healing your intestines.

Tip: Kimchi is a great dish to have with your eggs in the morning! You can add even more red chile flakes if you really like it hot.

Vary It! Omit the honey if you're doing the 30-Day Paleo Reset in Chapter 4.

Recipe courtesy Alissa Cohen, chef and author of Living on Live Food (www.alissacohen.com)

Vegetable Latkes

Prep time: 15 min • **Cook time:** 4–6 min • **Yield:** 5 servings

Ingredients	Directions
3 cups grated carrot, turnip, daikon radish, or zucchini **2 eggs, beaten** **Pinch of Celtic sea salt** **Pinch of pepper** **½ cup macadamia nut oil**	*1* Wrap a thin dish towel around the grated vegetables, 1 cup at a time, and squeeze out as much water as possible.
	2 In a bowl, mix the grated vegetables with the eggs, salt, and pepper. Preheat the oven to 250 degrees.
	3 Heat the oil in skillet over medium-high heat. Toss a pinch of the grated vegetable mixture into the pan; if it sizzles immediately, the oil is hot enough.
	4 Scoop ½ to ¾ cup of the grated vegetable mixture (slightly less than ¼ of the total mixture) into your hand and form it into a very loose patty.
	5 Set the patty into the hot pan and press it down gently with a fork. Cook at least 2 to 3 minutes on each side until nicely browned, keeping the cooked latkes warm in the heated oven. Sprinkle with a pinch of salt before serving.

Per serving: Calories 71 (From Fat 27); Fat 3g (Saturated 2g); Cholesterol 74mg; Sodium 125mg; Carbohydrate 7g (Dietary Fiber 2g); Protein 3g.

Vary It! You can add cinnamon to the carrot latkes, curry powder to the turnip, or fresh herbs to the zucchini.

Tip: If the oil starts to smoke or becomes dark in color, carefully discard it, clean the pan, and start fresh with new oil before frying any more latkes. Burnt oil is definitely not healthy or Paleo-approved.

*Recipe courtesy Mark Sisson, author of Primal Blueprint and Mark's Daily Apple (*www.marksdaily apple.com*)*

*This recipe has been vetted by the team at Whole9 (*http://whole9life.com*) and is considered acceptable for a cleansing 30-day Paleo launch.*

Lemon Cucumber Noodles with Cumin

Prep time: 5 min • **Cook time:** 5 min • **Yield:** 2 servings

Ingredients	*Directions*
1 whole cucumber	*1* Use a spiral slicer or mandoline to make pasta out of the cucumber. If you don't have a spiral slicer, you can use a julienne peeler or vegetable peeler and make thicker noodles.
1 whole lemon, zested and juiced	
1 tablespoon sea salt	
1 teaspoon ground cumin	*2* Place the noodles in a bowl and toss with the lemon juice, salt, and cumin.
	3 Transfer to a bowl and garnish with lemon zest.

Per serving: *Calories 39 (From Fat 5); Fat 0.5g (Saturated 0g); Cholesterol 0mg; Sodium 3,514mg; Carbohydrate 12g (Dietary Fiber 4g); Protein 2g.*

Tip: Double the batch for your lunch the next day.

*Recipe courtesy George Bryant, CEO and author of Civilized Caveman Cooking Creations (*http://civilizedcavemancooking.com*)*

*This recipe has been vetted by the team at Whole9 (*http://whole9life.com*) and is considered acceptable for a cleansing 30-day Paleo launch.*

Zucchini Pasta with Fire-Roasted Tomato Sauce

Prep time: 5–20 min • **Cook time:** 5 min • **Yield:** 2 servings

Ingredients

2 whole zucchini, peeled

Salt for draining, plus more to taste

¼ cup pecans, roasted

One 14.5-ounce can fire-roasted tomatoes

1 tablespoon coconut oil

Pepper to taste

Cooked Version

1 Use a spiral slicer or mandoline to make pasta out of the zucchini. If you don't have a spiral slicer, you can use a julienne peeler or vegetable peeler and make thicker noodles.

2 Place the zucchini noodles in a colander in the sink and heavily salt them. Let them sit for 20 minutes to drain all the water.

3 Pulse the pecans in a blender or food processor until you have small chunks — not quite a flour consistency.

4 Add the fire-roasted tomatoes and process on high to make a smooth sauce.

5 Preheat a sauté pan on medium heat and a saucepan on medium heat. Simmer the tomato sauce in the saucepan, covered, until hot.

6 Add the coconut oil to the sauté pan and sauté the noodles for 1 to 2 minutes to just warm them up. Transfer the noodles to a plate, dress with the sauce, and serve.

Raw Version

1 Complete Steps 1, 3, and 4 from the preceding Cooked Version recipe. Don't include Step 2 (the salting and draining step).

2 Plate the noodles and dress with the sauce.

3 Sprinkle with salt and pepper to taste and serve.

Per serving: Calories 217 (From Fat 144); Fat 16g (Saturated 7g); Cholesterol 0mg; Sodium 683mg; Carbohydrate 17g (Dietary Fiber 5g); Protein 5g.

Tip: This dish is a wonderful compliment to any protein for a complete meal, or you can serve it as a main course.

Recipe courtesy George Bryant, CEO and author of Civilized Caveman Cooking Creations (`http://civilizedcavemancooking.com`*)*

This recipe has been vetted by the team at Whole9 (`http://whole9life.com`*) and is considered acceptable for a cleansing 30-day Paleo launch.*

Chapter 17

Redefining Desserts

Who wants to go through the rest of their lives feeling guilty for indulging in sweet treats or even avoiding them altogether? Boring.

The truth is that you're hard-wired to want the sweet stuff; it's part of your natural design. What you aren't hard-wired for are the grain- and sugar-laden foods most people know as desserts. Most cakes, pastries, cookies, and other treats are refined-food overkill and become a burden for your body to deal with.

Luckily, every once in a while you can have your (Paleo-approved) cake and eat it too. You just have to redefine what sweets should be by using ingredients such as coconut flour, almond flour, fresh and dried fruits, nuts, vanilla, cinnamon, cocoa, honey, nut butters, maple syrup, and coconut milk.

Whether you go for the Blueberry Espresso Brownies, the Banana Cacao Muffins, or the Chocolate Ice Cream, you can relax. No guilt. The recipes in this chapter are super pure and super good! (The same can be said for the bonus recipe for Macadamia Nut Chocolate Chip Cookies you can find online at www.dummies.com/extras/paleocookbook.) ***Note:*** For all the recipes in this chapter, the serving size is one item unless otherwise noted.

Spotting Sugar in Its Sneakiest Forms

Wiping out sugar entirely is nearly impossible because all carbohydrates, even the healthy ones, are essentially sugar. However, you can control the *added sugar* and sweeteners in your food that provide no nutritional value.

Snub your nose up at these sugars and sweeteners:

- ✔ Agave
- ✔ All artificial sugars in boxes or packets
- ✔ Aspartame
- ✔ Brown sugar
- ✔ Corn syrup
- ✔ High fructose corn syrup
- ✔ Maltodextrin
- ✔ Molasses
- ✔ Raw sugar
- ✔ Rice syrup
- ✔ Sucralose
- ✔ Sugar cane
- ✔ White sugar

The absolute best way to reprogram your body to not reach for sugar or sugary carbohydrates is to go completely without sugar for 30 days. No cheating, no wavering — just 30 days of cleaning your body by getting rid of weak, unhealthy cells and building healthier cells for a stronger, more youthful body. The process is scary and difficult, yes, but I promise you it's one of those game-changers in life that's worth doing. I show you how in Chapter 4.

Cranberry Ginger Cookies

Prep time: 10 min • **Cook time:** 15 min • **Yield:** 20 cookies

Ingredients	Directions
2½ cups almond flour	**1** Preheat the oven to 350 degrees. Line a baking sheet with parchment paper.
½ cup almond butter	
½ cup unsweetened shredded coconut	**2** Combine all the ingredients except the cranberries and mix well with a hand mixer or stand mixer.
½ cup honey, melted	
¼ cup coconut oil, melted	**3** Fold in the dried cranberries by hand, ensuring they're evenly distributed.
1 egg	
1 tablespoon ground ginger	**4** Using a cookie scoop (smaller than an ice cream scoop) or two teaspoons, place scoops of cookies on the baking sheet, leaving room between the cookies because they will expand slightly.
½ teaspoon sea salt	
½ teaspoon baking soda	
½ cup dried cranberries	**5** Using your hand or the back of the scoop or spoon, slightly flatten the cookies.
	6 Bake for 10 to 15 minutes or until done.
	7 Remove from the oven and let the cookies remain on the pan for 1 minute before transferring them to wire racks to cool.

Per serving: Calories 133 (From Fat 81); Fat 9g (Saturated 4g); Cholesterol 9mg; Sodium 76mg; Carbohydrate 12g (Dietary Fiber 1g); Protein 2g.

Tip: These cookies will largely retain whatever shape you put them in before baking, so shape them as desired.

*Recipe courtesy George Bryant, CEO and author of Civilized Caveman Cooking Creations (*http://civilizedcavemancooking.com*)*

Almond Cookies with Cinnamon Glaze

Prep time: 10 min • **Cook time:** 20 min • **Yield:** 12 cookies

Ingredients	Directions
2½ cups almond flour	**1** Preheat the oven to 350 degrees. Line a baking sheet with parchment paper.
¼ cup coconut flour	
2 teaspoons baking powder	**2** Combine the almond flour, coconut flour, baking powder, and 1 tablespoon of the cinnamon in a mixing bowl and stir well.
2 tablespoons ground cinnamon, divided	
¼ cup macadamia nut oil or coconut oil, melted	**3** To the dry ingredients, add the oil, 1 tablespoon of the honey, the almond extract, and the eggs and mix into a soft dough.
3 tablespoons honey, melted and divided	
1 teaspoon almond extract	**4** Dust your work surface with more almond flour and lay the dough out, pressing to just shy of ½-inch thick all around.
2 eggs	
1 tablespoon ghee or butter, melted	**5** Use a biscuit cutter or the lid of a jar to cut the dough into circles; lay them on the baking sheet.
⅓ cup unsweetened shredded coconut (optional)	
	6 Bake for 9 minutes.
	7 While the cookies bake, prepare the glaze by mixing the remaining honey, the ghee or butter, and the remaining cinnamon in a small bowl.

8 Remove the cookies from the oven and brush them with the glaze. Bake for 9 to 11 more minutes or until done.

9 Remove from the oven, sprinkle with some shredded coconut (if desired), and drizzle the remaining glaze over your cookies.

10 Serve immediately or store in an airtight container for 3 to 4 days.

Per serving: Calories 121 (From Fat 81); Fat 9g (Saturated 6g); Cholesterol 31mg; Sodium 73mg; Carbohydrate 3g (Dietary Fiber 2g); Protein 9g.

Vary It! For a lighter almond flavor, substitute vanilla extract for the almond extract.

Recipe courtesy George Bryant, CEO and author of Civilized Caveman Cooking Creations (http://civilizedcavemancooking.com)

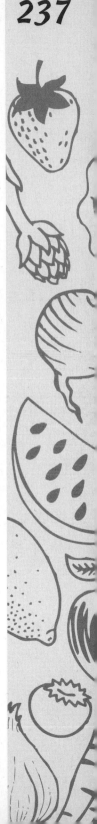

OMG Chocolate Chip Cookies

Prep time: 10 min, plus refrigerating time • **Cook time:** 10 min • **Yield:** 12 cookies

Ingredients	Directions
1½ cups almond flour	*1* In a large bowl, combine the almond flour, baking soda, and salt.
¼ teaspoon baking soda	
¼ teaspoon sea salt	*2* In a separate bowl, beat the coconut oil, vanilla, honey, and egg. Add the wet ingredients to the dry ingredients and mix well to combine.
2 tablespoons coconut oil, melted	
½ teaspoon vanilla extract	*3* Mix in the chocolate chips. Cover and refrigerate the cookie batter for 30 minutes.
¼ cup honey	
1 egg (room temperature)	*4* Preheat the oven to 350 degrees. Line a baking sheet with parchment paper.
¾ cup Paleo-approved chocolate chips	
	5 Roll the dough into 12 balls and arrange them on the baking sheet.
	6 Bake for 5 minutes. Remove the pan from the oven and flatten the cookies slightly with the back of a spoon. Put them back in the oven for about 5 more minutes, or until they look done. If you like soft and chewy cookies, take them out as soon as they start to turn golden brown.
	7 Remove from the oven and let the cookies remain on the pan for 1 minute before transferring them to wire racks to cool.

Per serving: Calories 134 (From Fat 72); Fat 8g (Saturated 4g); Cholesterol 16mg; Sodium 66mg; Carbohydrate 15g (Dietary Fiber 2g); Protein 2g.

Note: These cookies are so good that I gave them away for holiday gifts one year to rave reviews! They're a great way to introduce your friends and family to Paleo.

Note: If you aren't sure where to find Paleo-approved chocolate chips, try the Enjoy Life brand (available online at www.enjoylifefoods.com/chocolate-for-baking). They're dairy-, soy-, and nut-free.

Coconut Chocolate Chip Cookies

Prep time: 10 min • **Cook time:** 12 min • **Yield:** 12 cookies

Ingredients	Directions
½ **cup coconut oil**	**1** Preheat the oven to 375 degrees. Line a baking sheet with parchment paper.
½ **cup honey**	
4 eggs	**2** Microwave the honey and coconut oil in a microwave-safe bowl for 30 to 60 seconds to melt them together. Add them to a large bowl with the eggs, vanilla, and salt and mix well with a hand mixer or stand mixer.
½ **teaspoon vanilla extract**	
⅛ **teaspoon sea salt**	
1 cup coconut flour	**3** Add the coconut flour. Stir in the shredded coconut and chocolate chips.
½ **cup shredded unsweetened coconut**	
¾ **cup Paleo-approved chocolate chips**	**4** Drop heaping tablespoons of cookie batter onto the baking sheet.
	5 Bake for 12 minutes or until golden brown.
	6 Remove from the oven and let the cookies remain on the pan for 1 minute before transferring them to wire racks to cool.

Per serving: Calories 255 (From Fat 153); Fat 17g (Saturated 13g); Cholesterol 62mg; Sodium 43mg; Carbohydrate 26g (Dietary Fiber 5g); Protein 4g.

Note: If you aren't sure where to find Paleo-approved chocolate chips, try the Enjoy Life brand (available online at www.enjoylifefoods.com/chocolate-for-baking/). They're dairy-, soy-, and nut-free.

Tip: These cookies will largely retain whatever shape you put them in before baking, so shape them as desired.

Recipe courtesy George Bryant, CEO and author of Civilized Caveman Cooking Creations (http://civilizedcavemancooking.com)

Pumpkin Cranberry Scones

Prep time: 10 min • **Cook time:** 18 min • **Yield:** 12 scones

Ingredients	Directions
2 cups almond flour, plus more for dusting	**1** Preheat the oven to 400 degrees. Line a large baking sheet with parchment paper.
½ cup pumpkin puree	**2** Combine all the ingredients in a large mixing bowl and knead together with your hands.
½ cup dried cranberries	
¼ cup shredded unsweetened coconut	**3** Divide the dough in half. Dust your work surface with more almond flour and press half the dough out into a circle, about ¼-inch thick.
¼ cup crushed pecans	
1 egg	**4** Use a pizza cutter to slice the circle into equal wedges, making the pieces your desired size.
3 tablespoons honey, melted	
1 teaspoon sea salt	**5** Repeat Steps 3 and 4 with the other half of the dough and put the scones on the baking sheet. Sprinkle with a little more pumpkin pie spice or cinnamon if desired.
1 teaspoon baking powder	
1 teaspoon ground cinnamon	
1 teaspoon pumpkin pie spice	
½ teaspoon ground ginger	**6** Bake for 15 to 18 minutes or until a toothpick inserted in the center of a scone comes out clean.
	7 Remove from the oven and transfer the scones to wire racks to cool.

Per serving: Calories 177 (From Fat 117); Fat 13g (Saturated 2g); Cholesterol 16mg; Sodium 178mg; Carbohydrate 15g (Dietary Fiber 3g); Protein 5g.

*Recipe courtesy George Bryant, CEO and author of Civilized Caveman Cooking Creations (*http://civilizedcavemancooking.com*)*

Pumpkin Pie Muffins

Prep time: 10 min • **Cook time:** 20 min • **Yield:** 12 muffins

Ingredients	Directions
½ cup coconut flour	**1** Preheat the oven to 400 degrees. Line a muffin pan with paper liners.
2 teaspoons pumpkin pie spice	
½ teaspoon baking powder	**2** Sift the coconut flour and pie spice together. Add the baking powder.
¾ cup pumpkin puree	
½ cup coconut oil, melted	**3** In a separate bowl, mix all the remaining ingredients except the walnuts until well blended.
6 eggs	
2 teaspoons vanilla extract	**4** Add the dry ingredients to the wet ingredients. Mix well and divide the batter between the muffin cups. Sprinkle with the walnuts.
¼ cup honey, melted	
⅓ cup chopped walnuts	
	5 Bake for 18 to 20 minutes or until a toothpick inserted in the center of a muffin comes out clean.

Per serving: Calories 179 (From Fat 126); Fat 14g (Saturated 9g); Cholesterol 93mg; Sodium 57mg; Carbohydrate 11g (Dietary Fiber 3g); Protein 4g.

Recipe courtesy George Bryant, CEO and author of Civilized Caveman Cooking Creations (http://civilizedcavemancooking.com)

Cinnamon Chocolate Chip Muffins with Honey Frosting

Prep time: 15 min • **Cook time:** 18 min • **Yield:** 18 muffins

Ingredients	Directions
Honey Frosting (see the following recipe)	**1** Preheat the oven to 375 degrees with the rack in the middle position. Line a muffin pan with paper liners.
6 eggs	
¼ cup honey, melted	**2** Whisk or beat the eggs, honey, vanilla, butter, and applesauce in a large mixing bowl or a stand mixer.
1 teaspoon vanilla extract	
8 tablespoons unsalted butter, melted	**3** Sift the coconut flour, cinnamon, baking powder, baking soda, and salt over a medium bowl.
½ cup unsweetened applesauce	**4** Add the dry ingredients to the wet ingredients and whisk until well blended.
¾ cup coconut flour	
1 tablespoon ground cinnamon	**5** Fold in the chocolate chips, ensuring they're evenly distributed. Spoon the batter into the muffin cups.
2 teaspoons baking powder	
1 teaspoon baking soda	**6** Bake for 16 to 18 minutes or until a toothpick inserted in the center of a muffin comes out clean.
Small pinch of sea salt	
½ cup Paleo-approved chocolate chips	**7** Remove the muffins from the oven and let cool. Top the cooled muffins with Honey Frosting.

Honey Frosting

1 cup palm shortening

¾ cup full-fat coconut milk, chilled

¼ cup honey, melted

1 teaspoon ground cinnamon

Orange zest for garnish (optional)

Crushed pecans (optional)

1 Combine the shortening, coconut milk, and honey in a stand mixer or mixing bowl and beat on low for 20 seconds.

2 Scrape down the sides of your bowl and then beat on high for approximately 60 seconds until the frosting thickens.

3 Fold in the cinnamon and the optional ingredients (if desired) by hand, ensuring they're evenly distributed.

Per serving: Calories 265 (From Fat 198); Fat 22g (Saturated 9g); Cholesterol 76mg; Sodium 176mg; Carbohydrate 16g (Dietary Fiber 3g); Protein 3g.

Note: If you aren't sure where to find Paleo-approved chocolate chips, try the Enjoy Life brand (available online at www.enjoylifefoods.com/chocolate-for-baking/). They're dairy-, soy-, and nut-free.

Recipe courtesy George Bryant, CEO and author of Civilized Caveman Cooking Creations (http://civilizedcavemancooking.com)

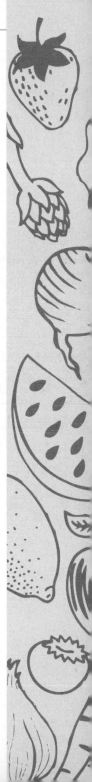

Banana Cacao Muffins

Prep time: 15 min • **Cook time:** 25 min • **Yield:** 9 muffins

Ingredients	*Directions*
2 ripe bananas	*1* Preheat the oven to 350 degrees.
3 eggs	
¼ cup honey	*2* In a mixing bowl, mash the bananas until smooth. Add the eggs, honey, coconut oil, vanilla, and almond butter and mix thoroughly.
⅓ cup coconut oil, melted	
1 teaspoon vanilla extract	
¼ cup almond butter	*3* Add the coconut flour and cinnamon and mix well. Let the batter sit for 5 to 10 minutes to allow the coconut flour to absorb the wet ingredients.
½ cup coconut flour	
1 teaspoon ground cinnamon	*4* Add the baking soda and chocolate chips. Mix until the baking soda is mixed through.
½ teaspoon baking soda	
2 tablespoons Paleo-approved chocolate chips	*5* Divide the batter among the muffin cups. These muffins will slide out of the pan without paper liners.
	6 Bake for 25 minutes or until a toothpick inserted in the center of a muffin comes out clean.
	7 Remove the muffins from the muffin pan and let cool.

Per serving: Calories 217 (From Fat 126); Fat 14g (Saturated 8g); Cholesterol 62mg; Sodium 95mg; Carbohydrate 21g (Dietary Fiber 4g); Protein 5g.

Note: Don't skip the resting time in Step 3. The batter will be too thin to scoop.

Note: If you aren't sure where to find Paleo-approved chocolate chips, try the Enjoy Life brand (available online at www.enjoylifefoods.com/chocolate-for-baking). They're dairy-, soy-, and nut-free.

Recipe courtesy Arsy Vartanian, author of Rubies & Radishes (www.rubiesandradishes.com)

Pumpkin Poppers

Prep time: 15 min • **Cook time:** 15 min • **Yield:** 20 poppers

Ingredients	Directions
Melted coconut oil for greasing	**1** Preheat the oven to 350 degrees. Use a little melted coconut oil to coat a 24-cup mini-muffin tin.
½ cup butter, melted	
5 eggs, beaten	**2** In a large bowl, combine the butter, eggs, vanilla, pumpkin, and honey. Add the coconut flour, salt, and spices (using ½ teaspoon of the cinnamon). Whisk to combine.
1 teaspoon vanilla extract	
½ cup pumpkin puree	
⅓ cup honey	**3** Let the batter sit for 5 minutes to allow the coconut flour to absorb the wet ingredients.
½ cup coconut flour	
¼ teaspoon sea salt	**4** Stir in the baking soda and then fill the mini-muffin tins with the batter until they're almost full.
1 tablespoon plus ½ teaspoon ground cinnamon, divided	
½ teaspoon ground nutmeg	**5** Bake for 15 minutes or until a toothpick inserted in the center of a muffin comes out clean. Tip the muffins out of the pan to cool on wire racks.
¼ teaspoon ground allspice	
⅛ teaspoon ground cloves	
½ teaspoon baking soda	**6** In a small bowl, mix the coconut sugar and remaining cinnamon.
2 tablespoons coconut sugar	
½ cup coconut butter, melted	**7** Dip the cooled muffins in the coconut butter and then roll them in the cinnamon sugar until fully coated.

Per serving: Calories 107 (From Fat 72); Fat 8g (Saturated 5g); Cholesterol 59mg; Sodium 70mg; Carbohydrate 9g (Dietary Fiber 2g); Protein 2g.

Note: Be sure you're using pumpkin puree and not pumpkin pie filling.

*Recipe courtesy Arsy Vartanian, author of Rubies & Radishes (*www.rubiesandradishes.com*)*

Chocolate Bacon Brownie Muffins

Prep time: 20 min • **Cook time:** 30 min • **Yield:** 24 muffins

Ingredients	*Directions*
2 cups almond butter	*1* Preheat the oven to 325 degrees. Line a muffin tin with paper liners.
2 eggs	
½ cup honey	*2* Using a hand mixer, blend the almond butter in a large bowl to make it a smoother consistency. Beat in the eggs and then the honey and vanilla.
1 tablespoon vanilla extract	
½ teaspoon sea salt	
1 teaspoon baking soda	*3* Add the salt and baking soda; slowly add in the cacao powder as you continue beating. Beat in the coconut milk.
¼ cup cacao powder	
2 tablespoons coconut milk	
8 slices crispy cooked bacon, chopped	*4* Fold in the bacon and mix well by hand to ensure it's evenly distributed.
	5 Divide the batter among the muffin cups and bake for 20 to 30 minutes or until a toothpick inserted in the center of a muffin comes out clean.

Per serving: *Calories 178 (From Fat 126); Fat 14g (Saturated 1.5g); Cholesterol 18mg; Sodium 142mg; Carbohydrate 11g (Dietary Fiber 2g); Protein 6g.*

Note: *Cacao* powder isn't the same as cocoa powder. *Cacao* is raw and unsweetened (much like a spice); it contains lots of magnesium and antioxidants. Cocoa powder is processed and contains cocoa butter to enhance flavor. I like Navitas brand (http://navitasnaturals.com/product/441/Cacao-Powder.html).

Tip: Cooking your bacon in the oven on a cookie sheet yields perfect bacon. Place the bacon in a cold oven and then set the temperature to 400 degrees. Wait 15 to 18 minutes, flip the bacon, and then cook for an additional 3 to 4 minutes.

*Recipe courtesy George Bryant, CEO and author of Civilized Caveman Cooking Creations (*http://civilizedcavemancooking.com*)*

Blueberry Espresso Brownies

Prep time: 10 min • **Cook time:** 30 min • **Yield:** 18 brownies

Ingredients	Directions
2 teaspoons coconut oil	**1** Preheat the oven to 325 degrees. Grease a 9-x-13-inch baking dish with the coconut oil.
1 cup coconut cream concentrate	
3 eggs	**2** Beat all the remaining ingredients except the blueberries in a large mixing bowl to mix well.
½ cup honey	
1 cup pecans, crushed	**3** Fold in the blueberries by hand so you don't crush them. Pour the batter into the greased baking dish.
¼ cup cocoa powder	
1 tablespoon ground cinnamon	**4** Bake for approximately 30 minutes. After about 25 minutes, insert a toothpick in the center and judge how much more baking time you need based on how clean it is.
1 tablespoon ground coffee or espresso	
2 teaspoons vanilla extract	
½ teaspoon baking soda	**5** Remove from the oven and let cool.
¼ teaspoon sea salt	
1 cup fresh blueberries	**6** If desired, drizzle some additional melted coconut cream concentrate over the cooled brownies.

Per serving: Calories 155 (From Fat 81); Fat 9g (Saturated 4g); Cholesterol 31mg; Sodium 75mg; Carbohydrate 19g (Dietary Fiber 1g); Protein 2g.

*Recipe courtesy George Bryant, CEO and author of Civilized Caveman Cooking Creations (*http://civilizedcavemancooking.com*)*

Pumpkin Brownies with Pumpkin Pie Frosting

Prep time: 10 min • **Cook time:** 35 min • **Yield:** 12 brownies

Ingredients	Directions
Pumpkin Pie Frosting (see the following recipe)	*1* Preheat the oven to 325 degrees. Grease an 8-x-8-inch baking dish or metal pan with the coconut oil.
1 teaspoon coconut oil	
1 cup coconut cream concentrate	*2* Beat all the remaining ingredients (minus the frosting) in a large bowl or stand mixer to mix well.
3 eggs	
½ cup honey	
½ cup pumpkin puree	*3* Pour the batter into the prepared pan.
¼ cup cocoa powder	
1 tablespoon ground cinnamon	*4* Bake for 30 to 35 minutes or until a toothpick inserted in the center comes out clean. (Start checking the brownies after 20 minutes to be sure you don't overcook them.)
1 tablespoon pumpkin pie spice	
2 teaspoons vanilla extract	
½ teaspoon baking soda	*5* Let the brownies cool completely before frosting.
¼ teaspoon sea salt	

Pumpkin Pie Frosting

4 tablespoons palm shortening	*1* Whisk or beat together all the ingredients.
2 tablespoons honey	
½ teaspoon vanilla extract	
½ teaspoon pumpkin pie spice	

Per serving: *Calories 193 (From Fat 117); Fat 13g (Saturated 8g); Cholesterol 47mg; Sodium 105mg; Carbohydrate 18g (Dietary Fiber 2g); Protein 3g.*

Tip: You can make these brownies in a mini-muffin tin — just reduce the baking time to 20 minutes.

*Recipe courtesy George Bryant, CEO and author of Civilized Caveman Cooking Creations (*http://civilized cavemancooking.com*)*

Maple Bacon Ice Cream

Prep time: 20 min, plus freezing time • **Yield:** 2 servings

Ingredients	*Directions*
One 15.5-ounce can full-fat coconut milk, chilled	*1* Combine the coconut milk, maple syrup, and vanilla in a blender until mixed well.
⅓ cup pure maple syrup	
1 teaspoon vanilla extract	*2* Set up your ice cream maker according to its operating instructions. Turn it on and pour in the coconut milk mixture.
3 slices crispy bacon, chopped	
	3 When your ice cream starts to solidify (about 10 to 15 minutes), add the bacon.
	4 Transfer the ice cream to another bowl and put it in the freezer for 30 minutes to 1 hour.

Per serving: Calories 620 (From Fat 477); Fat 53g (Saturated 43g); Cholesterol 12mg; Sodium 252mg; Carbohydrate 38g (Dietary Fiber 0g); Protein 7g.

*Recipe courtesy George Bryant, CEO and author of Civilized Caveman Cooking Creations (*http://civilizedcavemancooking.com*)*

Chocolate Ice Cream

Prep time: 20 min, plus chilling and freezing time • **Yield:** 2 servings

Ingredients	*Directions*
¼ cup honey	*1* Warm the honey and stir in the cocoa powder. Combine this mixture with the coconut milk and vanilla in a blender until the honey is fully dissolved. Chill the coconut milk mixture for 30 to 60 minutes.
2 tablespoons cocoa powder	
1 cup full-fat coconut milk, chilled	
1 teaspoon vanilla extract	*2* Set up your ice cream maker according to its operating instructions. Turn it on and pour in the coconut milk mixture.
	3 Let the ice cream maker work for 10 to 20 minutes, until the ice cream is partially set.
	4 Transfer the ice cream to another bowl and place in the freezer for 30 minutes to 1 hour.

Per serving: Calories 368 (From Fat 225); Fat 25g (Saturated 22g); Cholesterol 18mg; Sodium 18mg; Carbohydrate 41g (Dietary Fiber 2g); Protein 3g.

Recipe courtesy George Bryant, CEO and author of Civilized Caveman Cooking Creations (http:// civilizedcavemancooking.com)

Coco-Mango Ice Cream

Prep time: 10 min, plus freezing time • **Yield:** Five 1-cup servings

Ingredients	Directions
4 ripe bananas, peeled and roughly chopped	**1** Blend the bananas, mangos, and coconut milk in a food processor until smooth.
4 ripe mangos, peeled and roughly chopped	**2** Chop the chocolate into chunks your desired size and stir it into the banana mixture.
½ cup full-fat coconut milk, chilled	**3** Divide into 1-cup portions and freeze.
1.75 ounces at least 70 percent dark chocolate	**4** Remove the portions from the freezer 15 minutes before serving to allow them time to soften. (The low fat content compared to regular ice cream makes this ice cream freeze hard, like ice.)

Per serving: Calories 287 (From Fat 90); Fat 10g (Saturated 7g); Cholesterol 0mg; Sodium 8mg; Carbohydrate 52g (Dietary Fiber 6g); Protein 4g.

Note: Make sure your chocolate bar has no added soy or soy lecithin. Enjoy Life brand has a soy-free chocolate bar www.enjoylifefoods.com/chocolate-bars/.

Recipe courtesy Nick Massie, chef and author of Paleo Nick (http://paleonick.com)

Berries and Whipped Coconut Cream

Prep time: 20 min, plus refrigerating and freezing time • **Yield:** 6–8 servings

Ingredients	Directions
One 15.5-ounce can coconut milk	*1* Refrigerate the can of coconut milk for at least 3 hours (overnight is best).
2 cups fresh berries	
2 tablespoons sliced almonds	*2* When you're ready to make the dessert, place the can, a metal mixing bowl, and the beaters from a mixer in the freezer for 15 minutes.
1 teaspoon almond or vanilla extract	
2 tablespoons Caramelized Coconut Chips	*3* Gently wash the berries and pat dry with paper towels.
	4 Heat a skillet and stir continuously with a wooden spoon for 3 to 5 minutes, until the almonds turn golden brown. Transfer the toasted almonds to a bowl.
	5 Pour the coconut milk into the chilled mixing bowl and add the almond or vanilla extract. Whip on the mixer's highest setting until the milk is fluffy and resembles the texture of whipped cream, about 5 to 7 minutes.
	6 Divide the berries among four bowls and top each one with whipped cream, a sprinkle of toasted almonds, and Caramelized Coconut Chips.

Per serving: Calories 149 (From Fat 117); Fat 13g (Saturated 11g); Cholesterol 0mg; Sodium 17mg; Carbohydrate 8g (Dietary Fiber 1g); Protein 2g.

Note: You can find the recipe for Caramelized Coconut Chips in Chapter 10.

*Recipe courtesy Melissa Joulwan, author of Well Fed: Paleo Recipes for People Who Love to Eat and The Clothes Make the Girl (*www.theclothesmakethegirl.com*)*

*This recipe has been vetted by the team at Whole9 (*http://whole9life.com*) and is considered acceptable for a cleansing 30-day Paleo launch.*

Part IV

Paleo Slow Cooker Options and Kid-Friendly Dishes

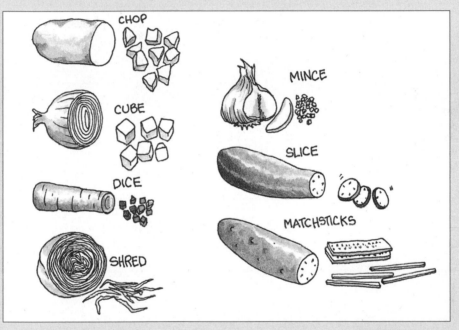

Illustration by Elizabeth Kurtzman

 If you're packing lunches for kids, head to www.dummies.com/extras/paleocookbook for great free ideas for healthy proteins and fats to keep them full and energized all day.

In this part . . .

- ✔ Choose minimum fuss and maximum flavor by putting your slow cooker to good use for one-pot Paleo meals.

- ✔ Entice your kids to help in the kitchen and learn about healthy foods at the same time.

- ✔ Leave your kids begging for secretly healthy foods presented in a variety of fun ways.

Chapter 18

Paleo Slow Cooker Meals

*B*ack in the day, before there were a gazillion prescriptions and medical treatments, people used slow cooked foods to get deep healing. Every nutrient was retained in the preparation, and the outcome was steamy, robust flavors. All the nutrition provided people's cells with the best raw material possible. It was natural healing at its finest. Getting back to using broths and slow cooked meals to help heal the body is a benefit of living and cooking Paleo.

As you prepare these easy yet decadent meals, know that you're giving your body simply the best. Bonus: Slow cooking is so convenient. You can cook your meals while you're at work, at play, or even sleeping. Now that's a good deal!

All the recipes in this chapter are Paleo perfection! Kalua Shredded Pork is an award winner, and the Sausage-Stuffed Peppers are just about the most perfectly balanced food you can find. The Deep Healing Chicken Broth can be the base of many meals.

Getting the Scoop on Slow Cooking

Whether you're a busy parent or just a busy person, do yourself a favor and get a slow cooker. Making meals this way is both convenient and wholesome. The slow cooker frees your oven and stove top for other uses, and it makes large gatherings or holiday meals so easy! Sauces and gravies cook really well in a slow cooker too.

Even at the low setting, internal temperatures of foods are raised well above 140 degrees, the minimum temperature at which bacteria are killed. If you're concerned about food safety, bring the food up to temperature by cooking on high for the first hour. (In most slow cookers, one hour on high is equal to two hours on low.)

Here are some general tips to get you fired up on slow cooking; be sure to also consult the user manual for your particular slow cooker model:

- **Working with a new slow cooker:** When using a new slow cooker, keep an eye on it during the first few uses. These slow cookers can have a mind of their own on high and on low — they can actually boil food, burn food, or just overheat — so don't leave one unattended until you have a better idea of its idiosyncrasies. Place the cooker on a cookie sheet, a granite countertop, the stovetop, or a similar surface that won't burn; the bottom can get pretty hot on some models.

- **Cooking fish:** Fish and seafood generally aren't good candidates for the slow cooker. If you use them, put them in at the very end of cooking, as with the Creamy Red Shrimp and Tomato Curry later in this chapter.

- **Cooking dense carbohydrates:** Cut Paleo-approved dense carbohydrates, such as sweet potatoes, carrots, squash, and turnips, into small pieces (about 1 to 1½ inches). In most dishes, you should layer these root vegetables on the bottom of the crock, under the meat and other ingredients, so that they begin to cook as soon as the liquids heat.

- **Browning meats:** Browning many meats helps reduce the fat content and can enhance the flavor and texture of dishes, but doing so isn't necessary. However, you should cook ground meats in a skillet before adding them to a slow cooker.

- **Using spices:** Stir in spices during the last hour of cooking. They lose their flavor if you cook them with the rest of the food or for a long period.

- **Stirring:** Try to refrain from lifting the lid to stir unnecessarily, especially if you're cooking on the low setting. Each time you lift the lid, enough heat escapes that you should extend the cooking time by 20 to 30 minutes.

Deep Healing Chicken Broth

Prep time: 5 min • **Cook time:** 11 hr • **Yield:** Six 1-cup servings

Ingredients	Directions
4-pound roasting chicken	**1** Rinse and pat the chicken dry. Place it in the slow cooker, season with the salt and pepper, and cook for 3 hours on high.
½ teaspoon salt	
¼ teaspoon pepper	
¼ cup roughly chopped onions	**2** Remove the chicken from the slow cooker and let it cool enough that you can handle it. Take all the chicken off the bones; refrigerate or freeze the chicken for future use.
¼ cup roughly chopped celery	
¼ cup roughly chopped carrots	
½ teaspoon dried rosemary	**3** Return the bones and skin to the slow cooker and add the onions, celery, carrots, and rosemary.
	4 Fill the slow cooker about two-thirds full with water (just enough to cover the carcass and bones, about 6 cups).
	5 Cook on low for 8 hours. Before using, strain the broth and discard the bones, skin, cooked vegetables, and rosemary.

Per serving: *Calories 20 (From Fat 9); Fat 1g (Saturated 0g); Cholesterol 0mg; Sodium 574mg; Carbohydrate 1g (Dietary Fiber 0g); Protein 2.5g.*

Tip: If you buy a precooked roasted chicken, you can skip Step 1 and prepare this recipe before going to bed to wake up to a beautiful, delicious broth.

*This recipe has been vetted by the team at Whole9 (*http://whole9life.com*) and is considered acceptable for a cleansing 30-day Paleo launch.*

Beef Bone Broth

Prep time: 10 min • **Cook time:** 10 hr • **Yield:** 12 servings

Ingredients	Directions
2 unpeeled carrots, scrubbed and roughly chopped	*1* Place all the vegetables and the garlic, bones, and bay leaves into a slow cooker. Sprinkle on the salt, drizzle with the vinegar, and add enough water to cover everything by 1 inch (about 13 cups).
2 stalks celery, including leafy part, roughly chopped	
1 medium onion, roughly chopped	*2* Cook for 8 to 10 hours on low.
7 cloves garlic, peeled and smashed	*3* Use a shallow spoon to carefully skim the film off the top of the broth. Pour the broth through a fine strainer and discard the solids. Taste the broth and add more salt as needed.
3½ pounds grass-fed beef bones (preferably joints and knuckles)	
2 dried bay leaves	*4* The broth will keep for 3 days in the fridge and for 3 months in your freezer.
2 teaspoons kosher salt	
2 tablespoons apple cider vinegar	

Per serving: Calories 285 (From Fat 126); Fat 14g (Saturated 5g); Cholesterol 78mg; Sodium 477mg; Carbohydrate 2.5g (Dietary Fiber 0.5g); Protein 36g.

Vary It! Feel free to substitute chicken, fish, or pork bones or to combine them all. Also, adding dried mushrooms or using 2 tablespoons fish sauce in place of salt (add it in Step 1) dramatically boosts the flavor of the broth.

Recipe courtesy Michelle Tam, author of Nom Nom Paleo (http://nomnompaleo.com)

This recipe has been vetted by the team at Whole9 (http://whole9life.com) and is considered acceptable for a 30-Day Reset Paleo cleanse.

Chicken Cacciatora

Prep time: 10 min • **Cook time:** 6 hr • **Yield:** 4 servings

Ingredients	Directions
1 medium white onion, sliced	**1** Line the bottom of the slow cooker with the onions.
1 pound boneless, skinless chicken breasts, halved	**2** Add all the remaining ingredients, pouring the tomatoes over everything last.
3 tablespoons olive oil	
1 large green bell pepper, seeded and sliced	**3** Cook on low for 6 hours.
1 large red bell pepper, seeded and sliced	
1 large yellow bell pepper, seeded and sliced	
2 cups sliced mushrooms	
1 stalk celery, chopped	
3 large cloves garlic	
1 teaspoon Italian seasoning	
2 cups chopped or crushed tomatoes	

Per serving: Calories 375 (From Fat 135); Fat 15g (Saturated 3g); Cholesterol 96mg; Sodium 391mg; Carbohydrate 21g (Dietary Fiber 5g); Protein 40g.

*Recipe courtesy Jason Crouch, chef and author of PaleoPot (*http://paleopot.com*)*

*This recipe has been vetted by the team at Whole9 (*http://whole9life.com*) and is considered acceptable for a cleansing 30-day Paleo launch.*

Mango Coconut Chipotle Chicken

Prep time: 10 min • **Cook time:** 4–6 hr • **Yield:** 4 servings

Ingredients	Directions
One 14-ounce can coconut milk	*1* Pour the coconut milk into the bottom of the slow cooker.
1 large mango	
1 pound chicken breasts	*2* Peel the mango, pit it, and cut the fruit into large and medium cubes. Add the flesh and the pit to the coconut milk (the meat on the pit adds flavor).
1 tablespoon dried chipotle flakes	
	3 Cube the chicken and add it to the slow cooker. Add the chipotle flakes and stir well.
	4 Cook on low for 4 to 6 hours.

Per serving: Calories 454 (From Fat 270); Fat 30g (Saturated 21g); Cholesterol 95mg; Sodium 94mg; Carbohydrate 11g (Dietary Fiber 1g); Protein 36g.

Tip: You can also use chicken thighs. If you can't find dried chipotle flakes, you can substitute an equal amount of red pepper flakes.

*Recipe courtesy Jason Crouch, chef and author of PaleoPot (*http://paleopot.com*)*

*This recipe has been vetted by the team at Whole9 (*http://whole9life.com*) and is considered acceptable for a cleansing 30-day Paleo launch.*

Easy Chicken Curry with Cabbage

Prep time: 10 min • **Cook time:** 4 hr • **Yield:** 6 servings

Ingredients	Directions
Two 14-ounce cans coconut milk	**1** Pour the coconut milk into the slow cooker and stir in the curry paste until dissolved.
3 tablespoons red curry paste	
1 to 1½ pounds boneless chicken thighs	**2** Cut the chicken thighs into 1-inch cubes and add to the slow cooker.
1 small yellow onion, chopped	**3** Stir in the onions and peppers.
1 medium green bell pepper, chopped	**4** Cut the cabbage half into quarters, and then chop each wedge into long, thin strips. Break the strips apart with your hands.
½ head cabbage	
	5 Stir in the cabbage, making sure it becomes coated with the curry mixture. (The cabbage doesn't need to be submerged in the coconut milk; it will cook down).
	6 Cover and cook on low for 4 hours.

Per serving: Calories 465 (From Fat 360); Fat 40g (Saturated 27g); Cholesterol 98mg; Sodium 798mg; Carbohydrate 12g (Dietary Fiber 2g); Protein 22g.

Tip: If you have extra cabbage, simply leave it on top of the curry mixture and it will cook down.

*Recipe courtesy Jason Crouch, chef and author of PaleoPot (*http://paleopot.com*)*

*This recipe has been vetted by the team at Whole9 (*http://whole9life.com*) and is considered acceptable for a cleansing 30-day Paleo launch.*

Pineapple and Mango Sweet Heat Chicken Wings

Prep time: 30 min • **Cook time:** 4 hr, 15 min • **Yield:** 8 servings

Ingredients	Directions
1 tablespoon coconut oil	**1** Heat the coconut oil in a large saucepan over medium-low heat.
2 jalapeño peppers, seeded and minced	
1 habanero pepper, seeded and minced	**2** Add the peppers and garlic and let them sweat down for a few minutes. Add the mango and pineapple and cook for a few more minutes, until the fruit softens.
4 cloves garlic, chopped	
1 cup chopped mango	**3** Stir in all remaining ingredients except the chicken. Reduce the heat to low and allow the sauce to reduce for 15 minutes
2 cups crushed pineapple	
One 6-ounce can tomato paste	
1 cup beef stock	**4** Blend the sauce in a blender or food processor until it's a uniform consistency, being careful not to let the hot sauce splatter.
2 tablespoons apple cider vinegar	
2 teaspoons paprika	**5** Set the oven to broil and arrange the wings on a foil-lined baking sheet. Broil for about 5 minutes per side, until they're just browned and crisp, working in batches if you can't fit all the wings on one sheet.
2 teaspoons cayenne pepper	
3 to 4 pounds chicken wings	
	6 Transfer the wings to the slow cooker and cover them with the sauce, stirring to coat.
	7 Cook on low for 4 hours.

Per serving: *Calories 691 (From Fat 387); Fat 43g (Saturated 14g); Cholesterol 167mg; Sodium 392mg; Carbohydrate 19g (Dietary Fiber 2g); Protein 56g.*

*Recipe courtesy Jason Crouch, chef and author of PaleoPot (*http://paleopot.com*)*

*This recipe has been vetted by the team at Whole9 (*http://whole9life.com*) and is considered acceptable for a cleansing 30-day Paleo launch.*

Kalua Shredded Pork

Prep time: 10 min • **Cook time:** 9–12 hr • **Yield:** 10 servings

Ingredients	Directions
3 slices bacon (no sugar added)	**1** Line the bottom of a slow cooker with the bacon.
1½ tablespoons coarse red Hawaiian sea salt	**2** Salt the roast evenly, massaging the salt into the nooks and crannies. Place the seasoned roast skin side up on top of the bacon.
5-pound Boston butt pork roast	**3** Cook the roast on low for 9 to 12 hours.
	4 Remove the pork to a large platter and shred with two forks.
	5 Taste to check for seasoning, using the cooking liquid to season.

Per serving: Calories 608 (From Fat 360); Fat 40g (Saturated 15g); Cholesterol 222mg; Sodium 1,438mg; Carbohydrate 0g (Dietary Fiber 0g); Protein 59g.

Note: Kalua is a traditional Hawaiian cooking method that utilizes an underground oven. This recipe lets you mimic it at home without digging up the backyard.

Tip: If you don't have red Hawaiian sea salt, any coarse salt will work. Keep leftovers of this dish handy in your fridge and freezer as an "emergency protein" for quick meals.

*Recipe courtesy of Michelle Tam, author of Nom Nom Paleo (*http://nomnompaleo.com*)*

*This recipe has been vetted by the team at Whole9 (*http://whole9life.com*) and is considered acceptable for a cleansing 30-day Paleo launch.*

Cheater Pork Stew

Prep time: 15 min • **Cook time:** 8–10 hr • **Yield:** 6 servings

Ingredients	Directions
2 small onions, thinly sliced	**1** Put the onions, carrots, and garlic in a 6-quart slow cooker. Season with ¼ teaspoon each of the salt and pepper and toss well.
½ pound baby carrots	
6 cloves garlic, peeled and smashed	
¾ teaspoon kosher salt, divided	**2** In a large bowl, combine the pork cubes, herb seasoning, fish sauce, and ¼ teaspoon each of the salt and pepper. Mix to combine.
¾ teaspoon pepper, divided	
3 pounds pork shoulder, cut into 1½-inch cubes	**3** Pile the seasoned pork on top of the vegetables in the slow cooker. Arrange the cabbage wedges to cover the top of the pork, drizzle with the marinara sauce, and add the remaining salt and pepper.
1 tablespoon any herb seasoning blend	
1 tablespoon fish sauce	**4** Cover and cook on low for 8 to 10 hours or until the pork is fork tender.
1 small cabbage, cut into 8 wedges	
1 cup marinara sauce	**5** When the stew is finished cooking, adjust for seasoning with the balsamic vinegar and/or salt and pepper to taste. Top with the parsley before serving (if desired).
1 tablespoon aged balsamic vinegar	
¼ cup finely chopped Italian parsley (optional)	

Per serving: Calories 639 (From Fat 297); Fat 33g (Saturated 11g); Cholesterol 195mg; Sodium 966mg; Carbohydrate 23g (Dietary Fiber 7g); Protein 60g.

Tip: Throw this stew in the slow cooker before heading to work, and a comforting, rib-sticking meal will await you when you get home.

*Recipe courtesy of Michelle Tam, author of Nom Nom Paleo (*http://nomnompaleo.com*)*

*This recipe has been vetted by the team at Whole9 (*http://whole9life.com*) and is considered acceptable for a cleansing 30-day Paleo launch.*

Pineapple Pork Ribs

Prep time: 10 min • **Cook time:** 6 hr • **Yield:** 4–6 servings

Ingredients	Directions
1 to 2 pounds pork ribs	*1* Cut the ribs as needed so they fit in your slow cooker and trim away any excess fat. Cut the pineapple into 1-inch cubes.
1 medium fresh pineapple	
2 tablespoons Spanish smoked paprika	*2* In a small bowl, combine the paprika, cayenne, mustard, and honey. Cover the ribs with this sauce as evenly as possible and arrange them in the bottom of the slow cooker. Top with the pineapple.
1 teaspoon cayenne pepper	
2 tablespoons sugar-free Dijon mustard	
2 tablespoons honey	*3* Cook on low for 6 hours.

Per serving: Calories 518 (From Fat 315); Fat 35g (Saturated 13g); Cholesterol 137mg; Sodium 227mg; Carbohydrate 16g (Dietary Fiber 1g); Protein 33g.

Tip: Choose leaner cuts of ribs, and the excess fat will simply cook off.

*Recipe courtesy Jason Crouch, chef and author of PaleoPot (*http://paleopot.com*)*

Meatloaf

Prep time: 10 min • **Cook time:** 4–6 hr • **Yield:** 8 servings

Ingredients	Directions
2 pounds lean grass-fed ground beef	*1* In a large bowl, combine the beef, eggs, bacon, veggies, oregano, pepper, thyme, 2 teaspoons of the paprika, and 2 teaspoons of the garlic powder.
2 eggs, beaten	
5 strips cooked bacon, chopped (no sugar added)	*2* Mix everything together by hand, forming a loaf that will fit into your slow cooker.
1 small white onion, diced	
4 scallions, chopped	*3* Place the loaf into the slow cooker and press it down so that the top is flat and you have about an inch of space between the loaf and the sides of the slow cooker.
2 stalks celery, chopped	
2 teaspoons dried oregano	
1 teaspoon pepper	
1 teaspoon dried thyme	*4* In a medium bowl, combine the tomato paste, mustard, vinegar, and remaining paprika and garlic powder; stir well. Spoon the mixture over the loaf, spreading to cover the loaf as evenly as possible.
4 teaspoons smoked paprika, divided	
4 teaspoons garlic powder, divided	*5* Cook on low for 4 to 6 hours.
One 8-ounce can tomato paste	
2 tablespoons sugar-free Dijon mustard	
1 teaspoon apple cider vinegar	

Per serving: Calories 293 (From Fat 153); Fat 17g (Saturated 7g); Cholesterol 119mg; Sodium 454mg; Carbohydrate 10g (Dietary Fiber 3g); Protein 26g.

Tip: For a spicy kick, add 2 teaspoons cayenne pepper to the meatloaf mix in Step 1.

Vary It! Ground chicken or turkey is a great option in place of the beef.

*Recipe courtesy Jason Crouch, chef and author of PaleoPot (*http://paleopot.com*)*

*This recipe has been vetted by the team at Whole9 (*http://whole9life.com*) and is considered acceptable for a cleansing 30-day Paleo launch.*

Sausage-Stuffed Peppers

Prep time: 15 min • **Cook time:** 6 hr • **Yield:** 4–6 servings

Ingredients	Directions
4 to 6 bell peppers, any color	**1** Cut the tops off however many peppers will fit in your slow cooker. Scoop out and discard the seeds. Poke a hole in the bottom of each pepper to allow liquid to drain out. Save the tops.
½ head cauliflower	
6 cloves garlic, minced	**2** Process the cauliflower in a food processor or blender until it's the size of rice. Transfer it to a large mixing bowl.
1 small white onion, diced	
2 teaspoons dried basil	**3** Add the garlic, onions, basil, oregano, and thyme to the cauliflower and mix by hand.
2 teaspoons dried oregano	
2 teaspoons dried thyme	**4** Add the sausage and tomato paste to the seasoned cauliflower and mix with your hands. Be sure to wash your hands thoroughly afterward.
1 pound ground Italian hot sausage	
One 8-ounce can tomato paste	**5** Spoon as much of the sausage mixture into the peppers as possible. Place them upright in a slow cooker and let them cook.
	6 Cook on low for 6 hours.

Per serving: Calories 295 (From Fat 162); Fat 18g (Saturated 7g); Cholesterol 37mg; Sodium 937mg; Carbohydrate 20g (Dietary Fiber 5g); Protein 16g.

Tip: To enhance the flavor of the sausage, lightly brown it in a large skillet over high heat and drain it before mixing it with the tomato and cauliflower.

Tip: Get the kids involved! Getting hands messy in Step 4 is necessary — a spoon just won't cut it — so let little ones have fun and help with dinner while you keep your hands clean.

*Recipe courtesy Jason Crouch, chef and author of PaleoPot (*http://paleopot.com*)*

*This recipe has been vetted by the team at Whole9 (*http://whole9life.com*) and is considered acceptable for a cleansing 30-day Paleo launch.*

Creamy Red Shrimp and Tomato Curry

Prep time: 10 min • **Cook time:** 6 hr • **Yield:** 6 servings

Ingredients	*Directions*
4 cups crushed tomatoes **One 14-ounce can coconut milk**	*1* Combine the tomatoes and coconut milk in a slow cooker.
3 tablespoons red curry paste **1 teaspoon ground cayenne or habanero pepper (optional)**	*2* Stir in the curry paste and cayenne or habanero (if desired). Add the vegetables and stir well.
½ head cauliflower, cut into large chunks	*3* Cook on low for 6 hours.
1 large yellow or orange bell pepper, seeded and cut into strips **1 cup chopped scallions**	*4* Add the shrimp to the slow cooker 10 minutes before serving. (Shrimp don't take long to cook, so don't forget about them.)
1 cup chopped celery **1 pound large uncooked shrimp, peeled and deveined**	

Per serving: *Calories 281 (From Fat 153); Fat 17g (Saturated 13g); Cholesterol 95mg; Sodium 1,364mg; Carbohydrate 21g (Dietary Fiber 5g); Protein 16g.*

Tip: You can use precooked frozen shrimp — just thaw and add to the pot a few minutes before serving.

*Recipe courtesy Jason Crouch, chef and author of PaleoPot (*http://paleopot.com*)*

*This recipe has been vetted by the team at Whole9 (*http://whole9life.com*) and is considered acceptable for a cleansing 30-day Paleo launch.*

Jalapeño Bacon Butternut Squash Soup

Prep time: 10 min • **Cook time:** 4 hr • **Yield:** 6 servings

Ingredients	Directions
1 large butternut squash, cubed (about 6 cups)	**1** Add all the ingredients to a slow cooker and stir well.
One 14-ounce can coconut milk	**2** Cook on low heat for 4 to 6 hours.
1 cup chicken stock	**3** Transfer the soup to a blender and puree before serving. You can also transfer the soup to another container and use an immersion blender.
2 carrots, peeled and chopped	
1 Granny Smith apple, peeled, cored, and cubed	
2 jalapeño peppers, seeded and minced	
7 strips cooked bacon, chopped (no sugar added)	
4 cloves garlic, chopped	
2 teaspoons Spanish smoked paprika	

Per serving: Calories 272 (From Fat 144); Fat 16g (Saturated 13g); Cholesterol 5mg; Sodium 151mg; Carbohydrate 32g (Dietary Fiber 8g); Protein 6g.

Vary It! Omit the bacon and use vegetable stock for a vegetarian version of this soup that's equally delicious.

*Recipe courtesy Jason Crouch, chef and author of PaleoPot (*http://paleopot.com*)*

*This recipe has been vetted by the team at Whole9 (*http://whole9life.com*) and is considered acceptable for a cleansing 30-day Paleo launch.*

Roasted Red Pepper and Sweet Potato Soup

Prep time: 10 min • **Cook time:** 4–6 hr • **Yield:** 6 servings

Ingredients	Directions
2 large sweet potatoes, peeled and cubed (about 6 cups)	*1* Add all the ingredients to the slow cooker and stir well.
One 14-ounce jar roasted red peppers in water, drained	*2* Cook on low for 4 to 6 hours.
One 14-ounce can coconut milk	*3* Transfer the soup to a blender and puree before serving. You can also transfer the soup to another container and use an immersion blender.
1 cup vegetable broth	
1 small yellow onion, chopped	
2 cloves garlic	
½ teaspoon pepper	
½ teaspoon red pepper flakes	

Per serving: Calories 199 (From Fat 126); Fat 14g (Saturated 12g); Cholesterol 0mg; Sodium 283mg; Carbohydrate 16g (Dietary Fiber 2g); Protein 3g.

Tip: If you're using store-bought vegetable broth, check the label for sugar, preservatives, soy, or additives of any kind. These are ingredients to avoid.

*Recipe courtesy Jason Crouch, chef and author of PaleoPot (*http://paleopot.com*)*

*This recipe has been vetted by the team at Whole9 (*http://whole9life.com*) and is considered acceptable for a cleansing 30-day Paleo launch.*

Chapter 19

Paleo Recipes Kids Will Love

1'm a mom. I have a business. I'm an author and just an all-around busy person. I truly understand the hurdles parents face to get their kids to eat healthy. At times, the task can be downright daunting, but it's a necessary one.

In 2004, the then-surgeon general asserted that modern U.S. children will be the first generation to not outlive their parents. This statement was a catalyzing moment for me. I knew I had to take action and make a difference, starting in my own home.

I've seen firsthand through my Superkids Wellness program that teaching children about nutrition and making them aware of healthier foods at a young age can have lasting effects. (If your kids are older, have no fear; as the saying goes, better late than never.) Have good food available and make it a part of your everyday life; kids absorb everything, and someday their understanding of the importance of nutrition just may surprise you. The recipes in this chapter (plus one for Make-Your-Own Cobb Salads available online at www. dummies.com/extras/paleocookbook) get you off on the right foot.

Packing Kid-Friendly Paleo Lunches

Taking the time to pack your kids (and yourself) a nourishing lunch is one of the best ways to set them up for optimal concentration. By thoughtfully combining foods in packed lunches, your kids will feel fuller for longer and be better able to concentrate on schoolwork and other tasks without being distracted by hunger or by blood sugar crashes.

Try to anchor your lunches with a high-quality animal protein. Protein helps you to feel fuller for longer.

Paleo lunch-packing is a matter of being able to easily pull from three sources: your leftovers, your fresh foods, and your nonperishables. Here are some great ideas from Audrey Olson of www.primalkitchen.blogspot.com on how to stay stocked up on all fronts.

✔ **Leftovers**

- Make double for dinner. This way, you always have at least a day's worth of leftovers to throw in everyone's lunchbox.

- Intentionally decide which night's meal will become the next day's lunch. This smooths your menu and grocery planning.

✔ **Fresh to-go options**

- Precut vegetables and fruit. Buy snack packs or cut them yourself and pack them in portion-sized containers.

- Buy single-serve store-bought packets of guacamole.

- Make a week's worth of Paleo quiches and egg muffins that you can easily grab and go.

- Pre-boil eggs for a fast protein option available throughout the entire week. You can eat them straight up or devil them (check out Chapter 10 for a deviled eggs recipe).

- Pack chicken, egg, or tuna salad (made with a Paleo-friendly mayo like the ones in Chapter 9) in individual containers or stuffed into peppers.

- Make DIY plantain chips or other homemade or dehydrated veggie chips.

✔ **Nonperishables**

- Put together small premade containers of homemade trail mix with nuts, coconut flakes, dried fruit, and so on.

- Consider jerky. Grass-fed beef jerky in particular makes a great option for high-quality protein you can toss into a lunchbox when you've run out of everything, including eggs!

- Keep individual packets of raw, unsweetened nut butters handy.

- Pick up dried fruits such as banana chips. Watch out for added sugars and other iffy ingredients, though!

Spiced Sweet Potato Fries

Prep time: 5 min • **Cook time:** 35 min • **Yield:** 6 servings

Ingredients	*Directions*
3 medium sweet potatoes	*1* Preheat the oven to 425 degrees. Line a baking sheet with parchment paper.
2 tablespoons coconut or macadamia oil, melted	*2* Cut the sweet potatoes lengthwise into ½-inch wide fries. (Each potato should make 6 to 8 fries.)
1 teaspoon garlic powder	
½ teaspoon garam masala spice blend	*3* In a gallon-sized zip-top bag, combine the sliced fries with the remaining ingredients. Shake vigorously for at least 1 minute to ensure that the oil and spices have evenly combined and coated each fry.
¼ teaspoon ground sea salt	
	4 Spread the fries evenly on the baking sheet.
	5 Bake for 35 minutes; check the fries to be sure that they're browning evenly.
	6 Serve the fries while they're hot.

Per serving (1 tablespoon): Calories 105 (From Fat 45); Fat 5g (Saturated 4g); Cholesterol 0mg; Sodium 130mg; Carbohydrate 14g (Dietary Fiber 2g); Protein 1g.

Tip: If you like your fries to be a little crisp on the ends, you can set your oven to broil and broil them for a couple of minutes after you check them for browning in Step 5.

Vary It! Garam masala blends usually contain cumin and other warm spices. Omit the garam masala if your family doesn't enjoy spicy foods.

*Recipe courtesy Audrey Olson, author of Primal Kitchen: A Family Grokumentary (*www.primalkitchen. blogspot.com*)*

*This recipe has been vetted by the team at Whole9 (*http://whole9life.com*) and is considered acceptable for a cleansing 30-day Paleo launch.*

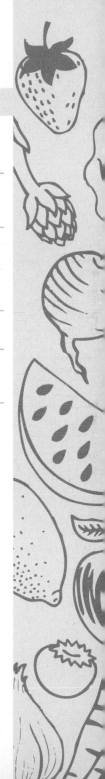

Barbecue Flavored Kale Chips

Prep time: 10 min • **Cook time:** 20 min • **Yield:** 2 servings

Ingredients	*Directions*
4 cups chopped fresh kale (stems removed)	*1* Preheat the oven to 350 degrees.
2 tablespoons cashew butter	*2* Wash the chopped kale, and then use paper towel to remove as much moisture as possible. Put the kale in a gallon-sized zip-top bag.
1 tablespoon bacon fat or coconut oil, melted	
1 tablespoon macadamia oil	*3* Blend the remaining ingredients in a blender or food processor until smooth.
2 teaspoons apple cider vinegar	
4 drops organic stevia extract (optional)	*4* Add the blended seasoning mixture to the bag with the kale. Close the bag and massage it for a couple of minutes to get the seasoning mix into as many crannies of the kale as possible.
½ teaspoon garlic powder	
2 teaspoons onion powder	
2 teaspoons paprika	*5* Spread the kale chips out on a baking sheet. Bake for 20 minutes, gently stirring the chips after 10 minutes. The kale will get a little limp before it starts to dry and crisp up during this process.
4 drops fish sauce (optional)	
Sea salt to taste	
	6 Watch the kale carefully as it approaches the 20 minute mark to make sure that it doesn't burn; you're looking for crispy chips that are dark brown on the edges, not black all the way through!

7 If needed, stir the chips and continue baking. If desired, finish the chips for 1 minute under the broiler just to crisp them a little more.

8 Enjoy your kale chips hot, fresh, and crispy straight out of the oven.

Per serving (1 tablespoon): *Calories 297 (From Fat 207); Fat 23g (Saturated 13g); Cholesterol 0mg; Sodium 694mg; Carbohydrate 22g (Dietary Fiber 4g); Protein 8g.*

Tip: Red Boat fish sauce is a premium fish sauce made with only anchovies and sea salt. It's a great addition to your pantry for this and many other Paleo recipes!

Tip: If you don't care for stevia but still want a little sweetness to your barbecue flavor, you can substitute a teaspoon of maple syrup or honey in your seasoning mixture.

*Recipe courtesy Audrey Olson, author of Primal Kitchen: A Family Grokumentary (*www.primalkitchen.blogspot.com*)*

*This recipe has been vetted by the team at Whole9 (*http://whole9life.com*) and is considered acceptable for a cleansing 30-day Paleo launch.*

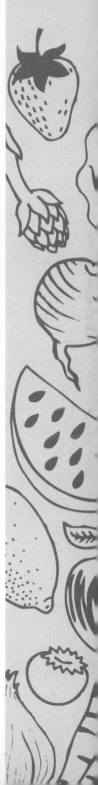

Lunchbox Stuffed Peppers

Prep time: 35 min • **Yield:** 4 servings

Ingredients	Directions
¼ cup Paleo mayonnaise	*1* In a medium bowl, combine the mayo, eggs, and relish. Season with salt and pepper to taste.
5 hard-boiled eggs, diced	
¼ cup unsweetened pickle relish	*2* Using a small spoon, scoop the egg salad into the peppers until just filled to the top.
Salt to taste	
Pepper to taste	*3* Enjoy immediately or save in the fridge for a future packed lunch.
8 mini sweet peppers, about 3 inches long, tops and seeds removed	

Per serving (1 tablespoon): Calories 192 (From Fat 126); Fat 14g (Saturated 3g); Cholesterol 246mg; Sodium 317mg; Carbohydrate 8g (Dietary Fiber 1g); Protein 9g.

Note: Chapter 9 has some Paleo-approved mayo recipes. Bubbies relish (www.bubbies.com/prod_pure_kosher_dill_relish.shtml) is one option for a live, lacto-fermented relish that is free of sugar.

Vary It! Substitute canned tuna in water or leftover baked chicken (diced) for the eggs.

Recipe courtesy Audrey Olson, author of Primal Kitchen: A Family Grokumentary (www.primalkitchen.blogspot.com)

This recipe has been vetted by the team at Whole9 (http://whole9life.com) and is considered acceptable for a cleansing 30-day Paleo launch.

Parsnip Hash Browns

Prep time: 15 min • **Cook time:** 15 min • **Yield:** 3 servings

Ingredients	*Directions*
3 parsnips, peeled	*1* Using a box shredder, shred the parsnips until you reach the core.
4 tablespoons coconut oil	
½ teaspoon ground cloves	*2* In a large skillet over medium-high heat, melt the coconut oil and then add the spices.
½ teaspoon ground nutmeg	
½ teaspoon ground cinnamon	*3* Toss the parsnip shreds into the pan. Stir and turn frequently. The parsnips will begin to brown, crisp, and clump together. Use a spatula to shape them into three hash brown cakes about the size of your palm.
	4 Continue turning the parsnip cakes for another couple of minutes, until golden brown and slightly crispy on the outside. Serve immediately.

Per serving (1 tablespoon): *Calories 274 (From Fat 171); Fat 19g (Saturated 16g); Cholesterol 0mg; Sodium 395mg; Carbohydrate 28g (Dietary Fiber 7g); Protein 2g.*

Note: Because parsnips are naturally slightly sweet but not overly starchy, this recipe is a palate-pleasing yet less-carby alternative to potato hash browns.

Vary It! You can substitute butter or ghee for the coconut oil. You can also try replacing the spices with garlic powder, onion powder, and salt before pan-frying for a savory take.

Recipe courtesy Audrey Olson, author of Primal Kitchen: A Family Grokumentary (`www.primalkitchen.`
`blogspot.com`*)*

This recipe has been vetted by the team at Whole9 (`http://whole9life.com`*) and is considered acceptable for a cleansing 30-day Paleo launch.*

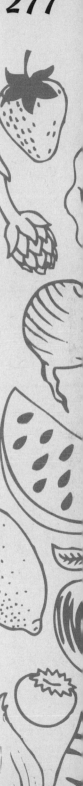

Sautéed Kale with Bacon and Mushrooms

Prep time: 5 min • **Cook time:** 10–15 min • **Yield:** 6–8 servings

Ingredients	Directions
6 cups chopped fresh curly kale, stems removed	*1* Wash the chopped kale and then use paper towel to remove as much moisture as possible.
4 tablespoons macadamia oil	
8 ounces mushrooms, cleaned and sliced	*2* In a large skillet, heat the oil over medium-high heat. Sauté the mushrooms, onions, and garlic for about 5 minutes, until the onions are translucent and browning.
1 large yellow onion, sliced into 1-inch pieces	
2 cloves garlic, sliced	
6 slices cooked bacon, crumbled	*3* Add the bacon and maple syrup to the pan and stir to combine, sautéing an additional 1 to 2 minutes.
1 tablespoon maple syrup	*4* Add the kale. Add the chicken broth ¼ cup at a time and cook until the kale is fully wilted, about 4 minutes. (Adding the broth gradually keeps the other ingredients from boiling.)
1 cup chicken broth	
Splash of balsamic vinegar	
	5 Drizzle with the balsamic vinegar, stir briefly, and serve hot.

Per serving (1 tablespoon): Calories 123 (From Fat 81); Fat 9g (Saturated 6g); Cholesterol 3mg; Sodium 156mg; Carbohydrate 10g (Dietary Fiber 1g); Protein 4g.

Tip: Adding bacon to cooked greens is a magical way to mask the earthy flavor of the greens and even inspire those you're serving to ask for seconds.

Tip: Substitute butter or ghee for the macadamia oil.

*Recipe courtesy Audrey Olson, author of Primal Kitchen: A Family Grokumentary (*www.primalkitchen. blogspot.com*)*

Raspberry Peppermint Sorbet

Prep time: 15 min, plus churning time • **Yield:** 6 servings

Ingredients	Directions
4 to 5 cups watermelon flesh, frozen solid	*1* Process all ingredients with ½ cup water in a blender until perfectly smooth.
12 ounces frozen raspberries	
½ cup unsweetened applesauce	*2* Pour the mixture into an ice cream maker and churn for about 30 minutes.
Pinch sea salt	
3 large fresh mint leaves, plus more for garnish	*3* Serve immediately; garnish with leftover mint leaves if desired.

Per serving (1 tablespoon): Calories 72 (From Fat 4); Fat 0.5g (Saturated 0g); Cholesterol 0mg; Sodium 50mg; Carbohydrate 18g (Dietary Fiber 4g); Protein 1g.

Note: If you don't have an ice cream machine available, you can serve the mixture just after the blending step. It makes this recipe a delicious and kid-friendly raspberry peppermint smoothie.

Tip: Four to five cups of watermelon equals about ten ice cream scoops full.

Tip: If you want the sorbet little firmer, put it in the freezer in another container for an hour or so. If you don't want seeds, you can puree the raspberry and then strain it before adding it to the other ingredients.

Recipe courtesy Audrey Olson, author of Primal Kitchen: A Family Grokumentary (`www.primalkitchen.blogspot.com`*)*

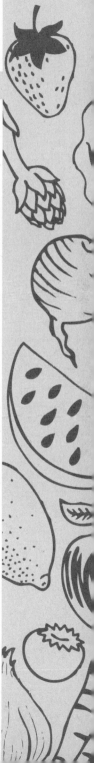

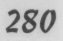

Raspberry Cheesecake Bites

Prep time: 45 min, plus refrigerating time • **Yield:** 8 servings

Ingredients	Directions
8 to 10 ounces dark chocolate, divided	*1* Melt half of the chocolate in a double boiler. When the chocolate is melted, stir it with a clean, dry spoon until it's entirely smooth.
⅔ cup cashew butter	
⅓ cup palm shortening	*2* Line 8 cavities of a mini muffin pan with paper liners. Spoon the melted chocolate into the cavities.
2 teaspoons apple cider vinegar	
½ teaspoon fresh lemon juice	*3* Let sit for 5 minutes. Reheat the chocolate in the double boiler and repeat Step 2 to thicken the chocolate base in each cavity.
¼ teaspoon ground sea salt	
⅓ cup maple syrup, or to taste	*4* In a large bowl, combine the cashew butter, palm shortening, vinegar, lemon juice, and salt. Using a stand mixer or hand mixer, whip the mixture until you achieve a cream cheese consistency. Beat in the maple syrup and vanilla.
½ tablespoon vanilla extract	
8 fresh raspberries	
	5 Spoon ½ teaspoon of the cream cheese mixture onto the chocolate in each cavity.
	6 Press a fresh raspberry into the center of the cream cheese mixture in each cavity. Top each raspberry with another ½ teaspoon of the cream cheese mixture.

7 Put the pan in the freezer for at least 30 minutes.

8 Repeat Step 1 to melt the remaining (previously unmelted) chocolate. Spoon the melted chocolate over the cream cheese mixture in each cavity; the melted chocolate should be level with the top of the cavity.

9 Place the pan in the fridge until the chocolate sets fully.

10 Remove the cheesecake bites from the pan and very gently peel off the paper liner. Serve the cheesecake bites within 24 hours of creation so the raspberries are at their juicy best.

Per serving (1 tablespoon): Calories 422 (From Fat 270); Fat 30g (Saturated 12g); Cholesterol 1mg; Sodium 80mg; Carbohydrate 32g (Dietary Fiber 1g); Protein 6g.

Tip: If you don't have a double boiler or don't want to mess with one, warm the chocolate in the microwave for 2 minutes at half power.

Vary It! Try other fresh berries (such as chopped strawberries or blueberries) or small pieces of fresh fruit in place of the raspberry. To make the bites nut-free, substitute unsweetened organic sunflower seed butter for the cashew butter. For sweetness without carbs, substitute a few drops of stevia extract for the maple syrup.

Recipe courtesy Audrey Olson, author of Primal Kitchen: A Family Grokumentary (`www.primalkitchen.blogspot.com`*)*

Star Fruit Magic Wands

Prep time: 10 min • **Yield:** 6–8 servings

Ingredients	Directions
2 large star fruits	**1** Wash the star fruits and slice them ¾-inch thick.
	2 Use a toothpick or steak knife to gently pry out any large seeds from the slices.
	3 Insert the pointy end of a bamboo skewer into the bottom of each star fruit slice, about 1 inch deep.
	4 Serve immediately or freeze for 20 minutes to create popsicle-style treats.

Per serving (1 tablespoon): Calories 7 (From Fat 0); Fat 0g (Saturated 0g); Cholesterol 0mg; Sodium 0mg; Carbohydrate 1.5g (Dietary Fiber 1g); Protein 0g.

*Recipe courtesy Audrey Olson, author of Primal Kitchen: A Family Grokumentary (*www.primalkitchen. blogspot.com*)*

*This recipe has been vetted by the team at Whole9 (*http://whole9life.com*) and is considered acceptable for a cleansing 30-day Paleo launch.*

Part V
The Part of Tens

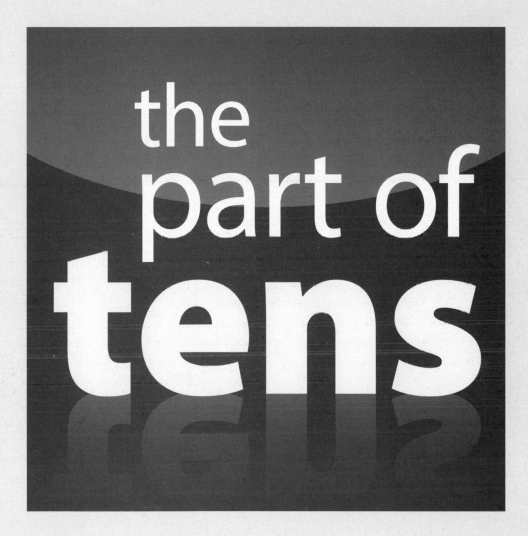

Compare what you think you know about Paleo cooking to some common myths debunked at www.dummies.com/extras/paleocookbook.

In this part . . .

- ✔ Make your life in the kitchen easier by picking up ten tools that are essential for Paleo cooking.

- ✔ Eat like a Paleo aficionado with ten favorite Paleo staples that you can use in meals or enjoy as snacks.

Chapter 20

Ten Favorite Paleo Foods

. . . .

In This Chapter

▶ Checking out great Paleo substitutes

▶ Focusing on nutritional powerhouses

. . . .

*I*f you're new to the Paleo lifestyle and wonder whether the food is boring, you'll soon find that eating Paleo is actually exciting. Some fantastic foods are a big Paleo yes, and this chapter gives you the inside scoop on these primal favorites.

What I love so much about these ten Paleo foods is that they're loaded with good stuff: vitamins, minerals, and antioxidants; Paleo-approved proteins; squeaky-clean carbs; and healthy fats. You can't go wrong. These foods taste great and have the *nutrient density* (lots of nutrients relative to their calories) to give your body the deep nutrition it craves. They're options that any true cave man or cave woman would love.

Organic, Unsweetened Coconut Flakes

Coconut flakes are a Paleo staple. What's so great is that they're a super-good-for-you fat. They're delicious on their own and one of my favorite travel foods; add some in a mixture of nuts and even some dark chocolate for a trail mix.

You can also sprinkle them on top of many dishes for rich flavor and some texture. My favorite place to add coconut flakes is to sweet dishes, such as on top of fruit (mango and pineapple are the best). Coconut flakes are one of those Paleo foods that after you buy them once, you'll always want to have some on hand.

I always call coconut the great wrinkle eraser. It has properties that heal the gut, and when your gut is healthy, your skin becomes radiant. It's better than any cosmetic cream you can buy in a jar.

Organic, Full-Fat Coconut Milk

Coconut milk is the meat of a coconut grated and squeezed to produce a milky product. It's perfect for replacing milk, yogurt, and cream in your diet. I also love adding it to specialty dishes like curries, creamy sauces, or soups; whipping some up to create a blissful whipped cream for plopping over fruit; and putting it in smoothies or drizzling it over berries for treats kids love.

Purchase organic, full-fat coconut milk. The organic stuff is healthier, and full-fat seems to work better in recipes. Always check the labels and avoid the brands with sulfites or sugar.

 Full-fat coconut milk is always sold in cans. With cans, you have to watch for BPA (Bisphenol A), which is a chemical used in consumer goods that has been linked to some pretty nasty stuff like cancer, infertility, diabetes, and heart disease. Here are some good coconut milk choices that are BPA free:

- Natural Value: www.amazon.com/Natural-Value-Organic-Coconut-13-5-Ounce/dp/B001HTI708
- Native Forest: www.edwardandsons.com/native_shop_coconut.itml

Almond and Coconut Flours

When I talk about my ingredient swap — that is, replacing non-Paleo pantry foods with Paleo-approved ones — I must say these flours always top the list. They replace traditional flours and grains used in recipes for baked goods, granola-type products, and even breaded coatings to make them Paleo-approved and avoid the I-swallowed-a-bowling-ball feeling those grains can cause.

 Just because these flours make your treats Paleo-approved doesn't give you license to load up on cookies and such regularly. Your Paleo template of proteins, carbohydrates, and healthy fats should still be the rule, with Paleo treats as the exception.

Organic, Pasture-Raised Bacon

There's nothing like the flavor or the crunch of a piece of bacon. Bacon appears in so many Paleo dishes — soups, stews, salads, wraps, seafood entrees, you name it — and can even be dipped in chocolate for a treat.

Here's what you need to keep in mind about bacon: It must come from a quality source. Get your bacon from an animal that was pasture-raised, and make sure the bacon contains very few other ingredients (no nitrates/nitrites, corn, wheat, or unnatural preservatives). Even better yet, go for bacon that contains no sugar.

The best bacon on the market comes from U.S. Wellness Meats: www.grasslandbeef.com/Detail.bok?no=1186. This bacon contains pork and sea salt only — no sweeteners, nitrites, or nitrates. Plus, it's Whole30 approved (see Chapter 4).

Organic, Cage-Free Eggs

Eggs are a Paleo staple that gives you what I call *flash protein* (a quick protein option). Whenever I travel, I almost always bring hard-boiled eggs for the trip.

Eggs are super versatile and are nutritionally just about the perfect food. They're filled with vitamins, including biotin, and minerals such as choline, which helps move cholesterol through the body. Flip to Chapter 6 for guidance on deciphering the labels on egg cartons to make sure you're getting the healthiest stuff.

If you have an autoimmune condition such as eczema, psoriasis, asthma, lupus, MS, Crohn's disease, or Type 1 diabetes, eggs may irritate your gut and create a sensitivity. If you're experiencing symptoms or flare-ups of these conditions, try omitting eggs until you heal your gut by eating other nutritious Paleo foods first.

Organ Meats

Before you say, "Yuck, organ meats?", hear me out. Paleo is about getting the deepest nutrition into your body in the most natural way. Organ meats are rich in protein, vitamins, and nutrients; liver, kidney, heart, and even tongue can provide you with a deep blast of serious nutrition.

Organ meats are an economical choice, but getting them from a pastured-raised — or at the very least, organically fed and antibiotic-free — animal is essential. The organs are what filter the pesticides out of the animal's body and can be quite toxic if you get them from a conventional source.

Bone Broths

Bone broth is a superfood on steroids. It's the healthiest stuff on earth.

Some people become concerned about getting enough calcium when they go Paleo because they're ditching dairy. Bone broth, though, gives you a whole new dimension of calcium. You get calcium *plus* a whole lot of minerals. The bones provide ultra-healing collagen as well. Throw in some chard, kale, collard greens, or spinach — all of which are also loaded with calcium — to make a gut-pleasing, calcium-rich meal. (You can find a bone broth recipe in Chapter 18).

Whenever anyone gets sick in my house, the first thing I do is make bone broth. It both heals acute problems such as infectious diseases and aids in the treatment of chronic problems such as cancer, diabetes, peptic ulcers, and more.

Sea Vegetables

The Paleo community has embraced sea vegetables, probably because they have tons of vitamins, essential fatty acids, and other natural antioxidants. They're particularly loaded with minerals, which every structure and function of the body depends on to function properly. Specifically, sea vegetables contain iodine, a trace mineral essential for healthy thyroid function.

Sea veggies taste kind of salty because they contain a balance of sodium and minerals from the sea, so they're a great replacement for salty snacks. You can also use them in dishes and as a garnish.

Here are my recommendations for sea vegetables:

- ✔ I love roasted, non-GMO SeaSnax seaweed and crinkle it into my meals almost daily: http://store.seasnax.com.

- ✔ *Kelp noodles* are a type of sea vegetable that tastes great in stir-fry; try Sea Tangle brand: http://kelpnoodles.com.

- ✔ This Emerald Cove brand dried sea vegetable blend is admittedly expensive, but it provides a nice blend of vegetables and is tasty: www.amazon.com/Emerald-Cove-Varieties-Vegetables-0-75-Ounce/dp/B001216DA2.

Sweet Potatoes

When you need dense carbs, sweet potatoes are such a comfortable place to go; they always taste great. You can dice them up in some beef or scrambled eggs, make them into a soup, or eat them on their own with some grass-fed butter or ghee. They're even sweet enough to make as a treat.

Sweet potatoes are the perfect post-workout recovery fuel. Some protein with some sweet potatoes will keep you well fueled and recovered after a workout.

I'm often asked why sweet potatoes are okay but not white potatoes. They both have nutrients, right? Right. But the peel of white potatoes contains a greater amount of *antinutrients,* which can create havoc in your gut and actually pull nutrients from your body.

Steve's PaleoGoods Snacks

Simplicity is key, and that's what you get with *Steve's PaleoKits* (http://stevesoriginal.com), a line of vacuum-packed snack mixes from Steve's PaleoGoods that are a go-to snack for many Paleo folks. They're perfect if you need a snack to carry in your bag, keep in your desk, or take with you when you travel.

All the kits are delicious and made with all high-quality, Paleo-approved ingredients. Steve's uses nuts, berries, and all grass-fed and grass-finished beef. The broader PaleoGoods line also offers PaleoKrunch cereal, PaleoKrunch bars, and more.

What I love most about purchasing from Steve's is that Steve uses the PaleoKits to fund his youth program, Steve's Club (http://stevesclub.org). Steve created this program to help get inner-city kids off the streets and give them a sense of purpose. Through leadership, CrossFit training, and dedication to nutrition, his club helps kids develop stronger bodies, minds, and spirits.

Chapter 21

Ten Essential Tools for a Paleo Kitchen

In This Chapter

▶ Making Paleo easier with time tested tools

▶ Creating a cave kitchen that works

*W*hen you have the right tools, any job is easier, and that sentiment applies to Paleo cooking. This chapter is a cut-to-the-chase guide to some equipment that has made my life — and the lives of many Paleo chefs I know — a lot easier.

Push aside your toaster, rice maker, and deep fryer and make way for ten essential gadgets that make healthy cooking a snap.

Chef's Knife and Sharpener

When you start eating Paleo, you prepare lots of meats and veggies; if you're like me, you want to chop them up with speed and accuracy. The chef's knife is an indispensable tool for that job.

The key to getting a good knife is finding one that you feel comfortable holding in your hand. It has to be sturdy and well-balanced with a broad, tapered blade. A 6-to-10-inch chef's knife is usually the best fit for most; 8 inches is a popular size. If your budget allows, you may want to look for a high-quality stainless steel knife because you'll be using it so much.

Cutting produces friction that dulls a knife's blade, so having a chef's sharpening stone is essential. To sharpen, slide the blade forward and across the stone with moderate pressure, keeping the blade against the stone at an angle. Repeat about ten times.

A great chef's knife on a budget is the Victorinox; it's a great value for the money. If you have a little more to spend, go for a product by Misono Guytou. You can score a decent knife sharpener for under $10 with AccuSharp.

Paring Knife

If you're going to do more delicate work such as slicing or peeling, you need a good paring knife. Anytime a bigger blade is awkward and cumbersome, a paring knife works brilliantly. It's really a natural compliment to your chef's knife.

You don't have to spend a whole lot on a paring knife. The key is to keep it sharp. My favorite paring knife is J.A. Henckels International Paring Knife.

Baking Sheets

Baking sheets are something that I use almost everyday. No, I'm not drowning my stress in cookies all day. I actually use the sheets to roast meats and vegetables and to make kale chips and baked Brussels sprouts, which I can't live without.

You should have two large baking sheets (about 13-x-18 inches) with rims; this size is ideal for roasting, baking, and catching drips when placed under other pans in the oven. Two smaller (6-x-9-inch) baking sheets with rims are great to have around for making some of the Paleo-approved baked goods. Plus, you have the convenience of fitting them into a dishwasher.

I'm a fan of stainless steel cookware. I avoid any coated nonstick cookware because of possible toxic fume exposure when baking at higher temperatures. And those nonstick surfaces almost always chip, which can leave bits of the coating in the food. I also tend to stay away from aluminum because high aluminum exposure has been linked to Alzheimer's disease. Keep in mind, though, that stainless isn't a nonstick surface, so you have to use parchment paper or a healthy fat like coconut oil to keep foods from sticking to the pan. I happen to like Norpro sheets.

Cutting Board or Mat

A large wooden cutting board is worth its weight in gold in your kitchen. Wooden cutting boards keep your knives sharp. My favorite cutting boards are by RedOnion Woodworks.

You may also want a small plastic board or a cutting mat that's easy to pick up so you can transport the food easily wherever you want it. Plastic boards are great for trimming meats and are easy to clean up.

Tongs

Tongs make life in the kitchen so much easier. You can't exactly use your hands all the time to flip and toss food. But you definitely don't need to spend a bunch of cash on this tool. You just need a basic pair of tongs with wide, scalloped pincers.

If you have room, consider getting a few pairs of locking tongs in different sizes. If you're doing a lot of high-heat grilling or flipping heavy foods, go for a pair by Progressive International.

Heat-Resistant Gloves

Everything in life evolves, and the oven mitt is no exception. You used to have to use a big, clunky oven mitt or a towel that was a huge pain to manage to avoid getting scorched by the oven or hot cooking vessels.

Now you have the option of *oven gloves*. These heat-resistant gloves look like what you would slip on to go outside on a cold day. They have five fingers and are made of a material called Kevlar or Nomex, which can withstand some serious heat (up to approximately 540 degrees). Ove' Glove is a popular brand.

Pots and Pans

Before you pull out your pans and get started, beware of using nonstick pans. As I note earlier in the chapter, the chemicals that give them that speedy clean surface are toxic, particularly if your immune system is compromised in any way. Stainless steel, ceramic, glass, and cast-iron cookware (preferably made in the United States or Europe) are safer, healthier alternatives.

Here are some of my suggestions for useful pots and pans:

- ✔ **Large deep baking pan:** Not to be confused with the rimmed baking sheet earlier in the chapter, this pan is great for roasting vegetables and making casseroles.

- ✔ **Large sauté pan:** A 12-inch sauté pan is perfect for sautés and stir-fries.

- ✔ **Large soup pot or stockpot:** You'll wonder how you survived without this pot. Get one larger than you think you need.

- ✔ **Large wok:** This piece is handy for when you want a quick, throw-together meal.

- ✔ **Small and large saucepans:** You'll use these pans for a number of dishes.

- ✔ **Cast-iron skillet:** This option is a heavy, durable pan that is a fraction of the cost of metal cookware. You can use cast-iron pans for frying, baking, or searing. They're super-efficient at conducting and retaining heat. Plus, they actually improve with age. If you're looking to buy a good cast-iron skillet at a reasonable price, I like Lodge Logic brand.

- ✔ **Muffin tins:** Mini- and full-size muffin tins are great additions to your kitchen. I'm excited that I can now find cast-iron muffin tins that can make Paleo muffins without fail (in full-size, at least; I still haven't been able to get my hands on cast-iron mini-muffin tins).

Meat Thermometer

Every Paleo kitchen should be equipped with a good meat thermometer. If you've ever had to cut into a roast or a turkey to see whether it's done or have paid a fortune for good meat only to end up overcooking it, then you know what I'm saying. If nothing else, a meat thermometer is great for just making sure your meats are cooked at a safe temperature to prevent food-borne illnesses.

I like instant-read probe thermometers. They have a display that sits outside the oven. You just stick the probe into the center of the meat, make sure it's plugged into the display, and roast until the meat reaches the desired internal temperature. It's convenient, accurate, and inexpensive. Invest in a good thermometer so you get an accurate read: The Digital In-Oven Thermometer and Timer by Polder does the trick nicely.

Mixing Bowls

Mixing bowls are a kitchen must-have. I prefer stainless steel mixing bowls. They clean up nicely, you can put them in the dishwasher, and they won't break on granite countertops, which can happen to glass bowls. Look for the kind that has a rubber bottom, which prevents the bowl from sliding when you're trying to stir. Some even come with a plastic lid, which allows you store your food and makes for easy transport.

I recommend having at least three or four different sizes of bowls. When you're baking or cooking, you may have to mix different sets of ingredients in separate bowls or keep track of more than one cooking project at once. Plus, you may have some bowls that are being occupied already, storing your foods from previous meals. Luckily, most bowls come in stackable sets, which take up less storage space.

They may be expensive, but MUI France makes a killer set of bowls that will last forever and grip the countertop well.

Small Tools and Gadgets

Everyone loves gadgets. In the kitchen, you can get particularly crazy because these gadgets make delving into recipes fun and smooth going. Here are a few small essentials:

- ✔ **Zester:** A citrus zester is valuable because adding zest to your meals is an easy way to add flavor and nutrition without extra calories or other additives.

- ✔ **Immersion blenders:** These hand-held blenders are, well, handy anytime you want to blend something up quickly and without a mess. The biggest bonus is the ability to blend food right in the pot.

- ✔ **Julienne peeler:** A julienne peeler works like a charm for turning vegetables such zucchini and summer squash into faux noodles for lasagna and pasta.

- ✔ **Whisk:** A whisk is nice to have available when you want to whip something up quickly, such as a wonderful whipped coconut cream or an egg mixture for an omelet.

- ✔ **Wooden spatula:** You can use wooden spatulas for almost everything you stir and mix in the kitchen. The wood is ideal for sensitive surfaces on your cookware.

Appendix

Metric Conversion Guide

· ·

*N*ote: The recipes in this book weren't developed or tested using metric measurements. There may be some variation in quality when converting to metric units.

Common Abbreviations

Abbreviation(s)	What It Stands For
cm	Centimeter
C., c.	Cup
G, g	Gram
kg	Kilogram
L, l	Liter
lb.	Pound
mL, ml	Milliliter
oz.	Ounce
pt.	Pint
t., tsp.	Teaspoon
T., Tb., Tbsp.	Tablespoon

Volume

U.S. Units	Canadian Metric	Australian Metric
¼ teaspoon	1 milliliter	1 milliliter
½ teaspoon	2 milliliters	2 milliliters
1 teaspoon	5 milliliters	5 milliliters
1 tablespoon	15 milliliters	20 milliliters

(continued)

Volume *(continued)*

U.S. Units	Canadian Metric	Australian Metric
¼ cup	50 milliliters	60 milliliters
⅓ cup	75 milliliters	80 milliliters
½ cup	125 milliliters	125 milliliters
⅔ cup	150 milliliters	170 milliliters
¾ cup	175 milliliters	190 milliliters
1 cup	250 milliliters	250 milliliters
1 quart	1 liter	1 liter
1½ quarts	1.5 liters	1.5 liters
2 quarts	2 liters	2 liters
2½ quarts	2.5 liters	2.5 liters
3 quarts	3 liters	3 liters
4 quarts (1 gallon)	4 liters	4 liters

Weight

U.S. Units	Canadian Metric	Australian Metric
1 ounce	30 grams	30 grams
2 ounces	55 grams	60 grams
3 ounces	85 grams	90 grams
4 ounces (¼ pound)	115 grams	125 grams
8 ounces (½ pound)	225 grams	225 grams
16 ounces (1 pound)	455 grams	500 grams (½ kilogram)

Length

Inches	Centimeters
0.5	1.5
1	2.5
2	5.0
3	7.5

Inches	Centimeters
4	10.0
5	12.5
6	15.0
7	17.5
8	20.5
9	23.0
10	25.5
11	28.0
12	30.5

Temperature (Degrees)

Fahrenheit	Celsius
32	0
212	100
250	120
275	140
300	150
325	160
350	180
375	190
400	200
425	220
450	230
475	240
500	260

Index

About the Author

Dr. Kellyann Petrucci earned her BA from Temple University, hosted her alma mater's Department of Public Health Intern Program, and mentored students entering the health field. She earned her MS degree from St. Joseph's University and her Doctor of Chiropractic degree from Logan College of Chiropractic/University Programs, where she served as the postgraduate chairperson. Dr. Kellyann did postgraduate coursework in Europe. She studied Naturopathic Medicine at the College of Naturopathic Medicine in London, and she is one of the few practitioners in the United States certified in biological medicine by the esteemed Dr. Thomas Rau of the Paracelsus Klinik Lustmuhle in Switzerland.

In Dr. Kellyann's many years of thriving nutritional based practice and consulting, she helped patients build the strongest healthiest body possible. She learned early on that looking and feeling amazing came down to learning simple principles and food values that made astonishing differences in people's lives. She realized that deep nutrition wasn't about fancy powders, ancient elixirs, or the latest creams; it was about reprogramming your body to get back to the basics and eat the way you were designed. She found the principles of living Paleo to be the key for people who want to lose weight, boost immunity, and fight aging. Dr. Kellyann has seen so much success from those eating Paleo that she feels a moral obligation to spread the message of eating real food.

Dr. Kellyann is the coauthor for the health and lifestyle books *Living Paleo For Dummies* and *Boosting Your Immunity For Dummies* (both from Wiley). She also created the successful kids' health and wellness program Superkids Wellness and the Paleo door-to-door home delivery food service Living Paleo Foods (www.livingpaleofoods.com). You can find free nutritional videos, tips and recipes, and her latest news segments on her website, DrKellyann.com (http://drkellyann.com). Look her up on Twitter as @drkellyann.

Dedication

Those who know me know I love to eat. This passion is second, though, to my love affair for sharing thoughts, ideas, memories, and laughs over a meal.

I dedicate this book to everyone I've ever shared a table with. Whether it was in finest restaurant in Paris or the local diner, that meal — that experience — will always be a part of my life's story.

I dedicate Chapter 4 in particular to Melissa and Dallas Hartwig, New York Times best-selling authors of *It Starts With Food* (Victory Belt Publishing) and the popular website whole9life (http://whole9life.com). They're the messengers who inspired the 30-Day Reset. I'm immensely in awe of their nonstop commitment and undaunted passion to make the world a healthier place.

And to my beautiful boys, who had to endure my empty chair at the table more than once during my marathon year of writing. You are my "why," and having you in my life is what generates every bit of my power.

Salute!

Author's Acknowledgments

A super big hug and deep respect goes to my fabulous contributors, all of whom are some of the best and brightest chefs and recipe bloggers — and now my friends. Thanks for sharing your mouth-watering gifts and being such a pleasure to work with: Melissa Joulwan of www.theclothes makethegirl.com; Michelle Tam of http://nomnompaleo.com; Mark Sisson of www.marksdailyapple.com; Arsy Vartanian of www. rubiesandradishes.com; George Bryant of http://civilized cavemancooking.com; Nick Massie of www.paleonick.com; Jason Crouch of www.paleopot.com; Audrey Olson of http://primalkitchen. blogspot.com; and Alissa Cohen of www.alissacohen.com.

If anyone has ever given you a shot in life, you'll know why I have such deep gratitude for my agent, Bill Gladstone of Waterside Productions. He gave me my first big break purely from instinct, and I am forever thankful for his faith and intuition. To Margot Hutchinson of Waterside Productions, who was on my side pitching from the beginning and who is now more than my agent; she has become special in my life.

To my colleagues at Wiley, especially Senior Acquisitions Editor Tracy Boggier, who is one of those people who has a million things to do and a million fires going on around her and still gets it all done with grace. Thanks for always being so good to me. To my Project Editor, Elizabeth Rea, who is the most organized person I have ever met in my life. Thanks for lending your talents (once again) to help me build a beautiful book. Copy Editor Megan Knoll always adds awesome perspective and quality. And to my Technical Reviewer Amy Kubal, it was an honor to have your watchful eye. Amy is so well seasoned and has such deep knowledge in living Paleo, this book can't help but be spot on. Thanks for everything, Amy!

Publisher's Acknowledgments

Senior Acquisitions Editor: Tracy Boggier

Project Editor: Elizabeth Rea

Copy Editor: Megan Knoll

Technical Editor: Amy Kubal, MS, RD, LN

Art Coordinator: Alicia B. South

Project Coordinator: Sheree Montgomery

Food Photographer: T.J. Hine

Food Stylist: Lisa Bishop

Illustrator: Elizabeth Kurtzman

Cover Images: T.J. Hine Photography

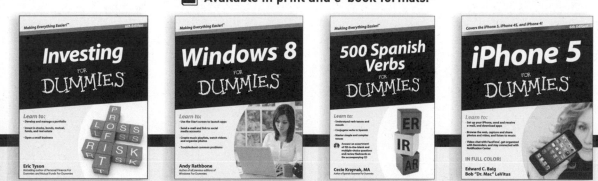

Math & Science

Algebra I For Dummies,
2nd Edition
978-0-470-55964-2

Anatomy and Physiology
For Dummies,
2nd Edition
978-0-470-92326-9

Astronomy For Dummies,
3rd Edition
978-1-118-37697-3

Biology For Dummies,
2nd Edition
978-0-470-59875-7

Chemistry For Dummies,
2nd Edition
978-1-1180-0730-3

Pre-Algebra Essentials
For Dummies
978-0-470-61838-7

Microsoft Office

Excel 2013 For Dummies
978-1-118-51012-4

Office 2013 All-in-One
For Dummies
978-1-118-51636-2

PowerPoint 2013
For Dummies
978-1-118-50253-2

Word 2013 For Dummies
978-1-118-49123-2

Music

Blues Harmonica
For Dummies
978-1-118-25269-7

Guitar For Dummies,
3rd Edition
978-1-118-11554-1

iPod & iTunes
For Dummies,
10th Edition
978-1-118-50864-0

Programming

Android Application
Development For
Dummies, 2nd Edition
978-1-118-38710-8

iOS 6 Application
Development For Dummies
978-1-118-50880-0

Java For Dummies,
5th Edition
978-0-470-37173-2

Religion & Inspiration

The Bible For Dummies
978-0-7645-5296-0

Buddhism For Dummies,
2nd Edition
978-1-118-02379-2

Catholicism For Dummies,
2nd Edition
978-1-118-07778-8

Self-Help & Relationships

Bipolar Disorder
For Dummies,
2nd Edition
978-1-118-33882-7

Meditation For Dummies,
3rd Edition
978-1-118-29144-3

Seniors

Computers For Seniors
For Dummies,
3rd Edition
978-1-118-11553-4

iPad For Seniors
For Dummies,
5th Edition
978-1-118-49708-1

Social Security
For Dummies
978-1-118-20573-0

Smartphones & Tablets

Android Phones
For Dummies
978-1-118-16952-0

Kindle Fire HD
For Dummies
978-1-118-42223-6

NOOK HD For Dummies,
Portable Edition
978-1-118-39498-4

Surface For Dummies
978-1-118-49634-3

Test Prep

ACT For Dummies,
5th Edition
978-1-118-01259-8

ASVAB For Dummies,
3rd Edition
978-0-470-63760-9

GRE For Dummies,
7th Edition
978-0-470-88921-3

Officer Candidate Tests,
For Dummies
978-0-470-59876-4

Physician's Assistant Exa
For Dummies
978-1-118-11556-5

Series 7 Exam
For Dummies
978-0-470-09932-2

Windows 8

Windows 8 For Dummies
978-1-118-13461-0

Windows 8 For Dummies
Book + DVD Bundle
978-1-118-27167-4

Windows 8 All-in-One
For Dummies
978-1-118-11920-4

Available in print and e-book formats.

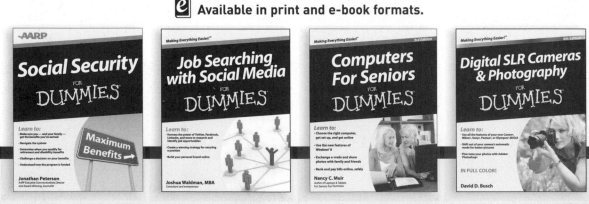

Available wherever books are sold. For more information or to order direct: U.S. customers visit www.Dummies.com or call 1-877-762-2
U.K. customers visit www.Wileyeurope.com or call (0) 1243 843291. Canadian customers visit www.Wiley.ca or call 1-800-567-4797.

Connect with us online at www.facebook.com/fordummies or @fordummies

Take Dummies with you everywhere you go!

Whether you're excited about e-books, want more from the web, must have your mobile apps, or swept up in social media, Dummies makes everything easier .

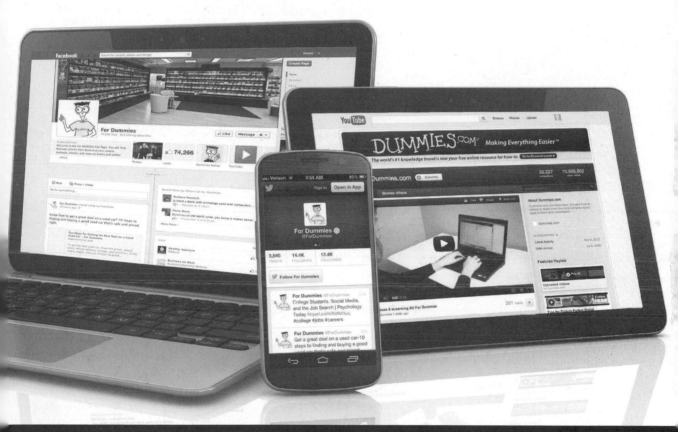

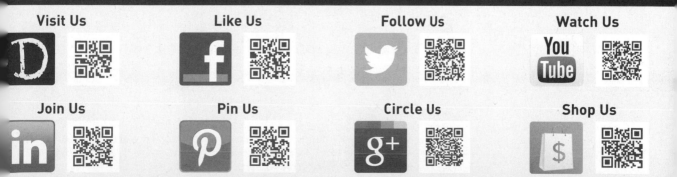

Dummies products make life easier

- DIY
- Consumer Electronics
- Crafts
- Software
- Cookware
- Hobbies
- Videos
- Music
- Games
- and More!

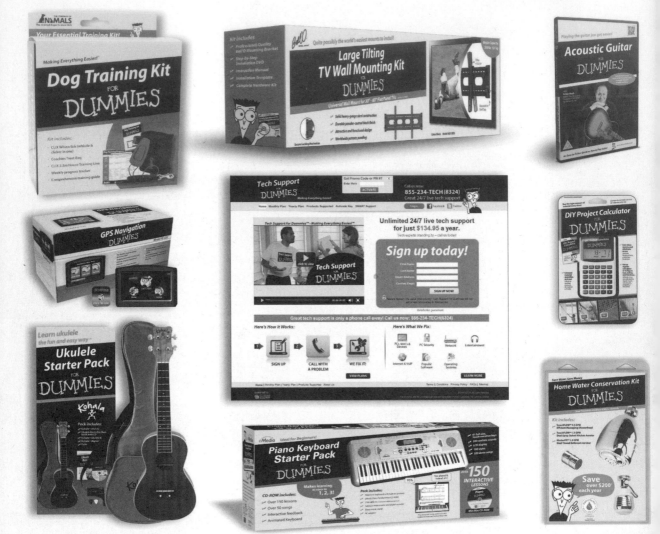

For more information, go to **Dummies.com**® and search the store by category.

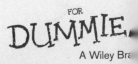

FOR
DUMMIE.
A Wiley Bra